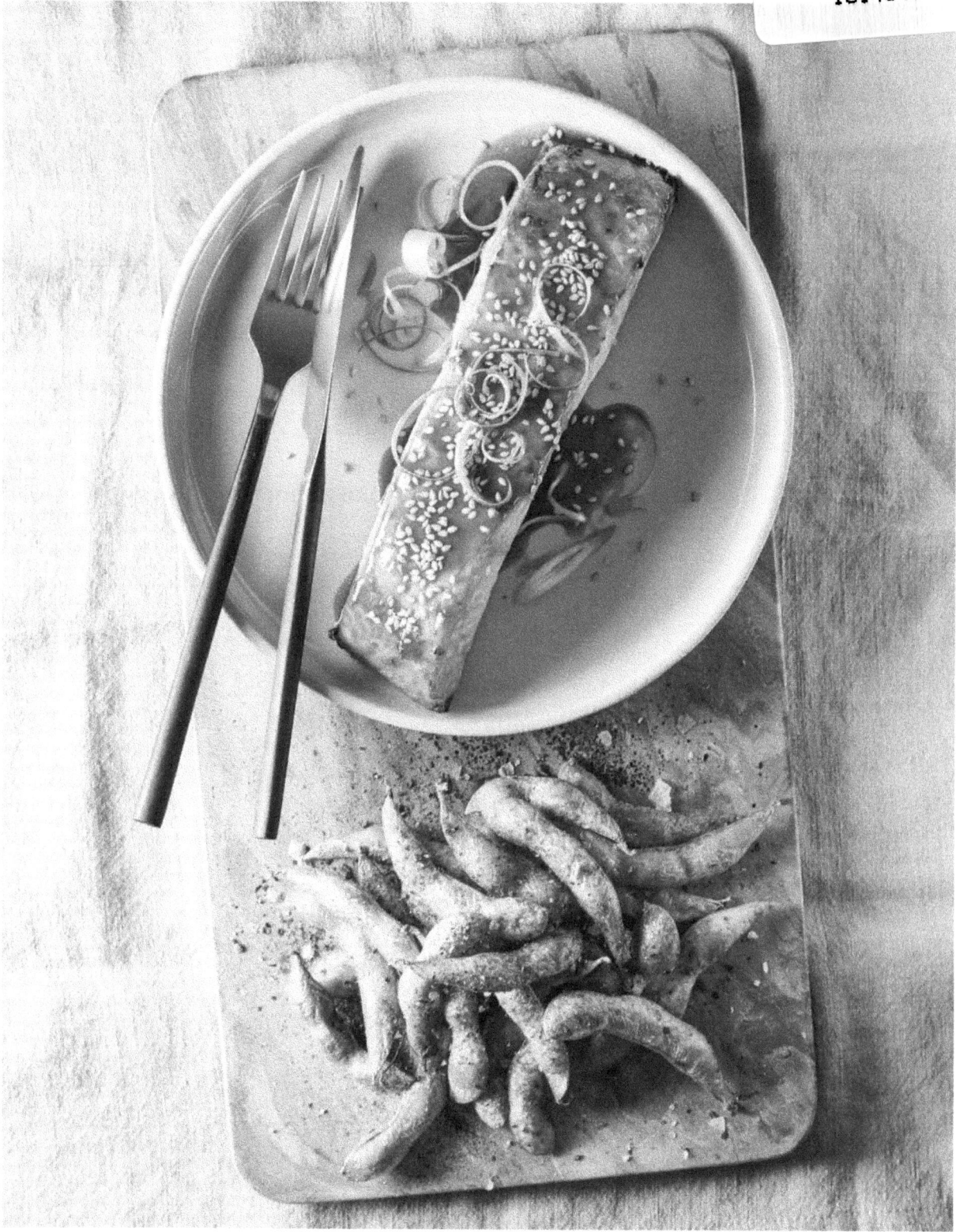

AIR FRYER COOKBOOK

for Weight Loss

100 Easy and Delicious recipes to make at home every day

Photography © 2020 Marija Vidal. Food styling by Elisabet der Nederlanden.

Cover: Maryland-Style Crab Cakes

ISBN: Print 978-1-64611-894-6 | eBook 978-1-64611-895-3

R0

To my loving husband, Daniel, who pushed me past my comfort zone to go after my dreams. And to my children, Gabriel, Jaiden, Avery, and Emersyn, who captured my heart with the first beats of theirs.

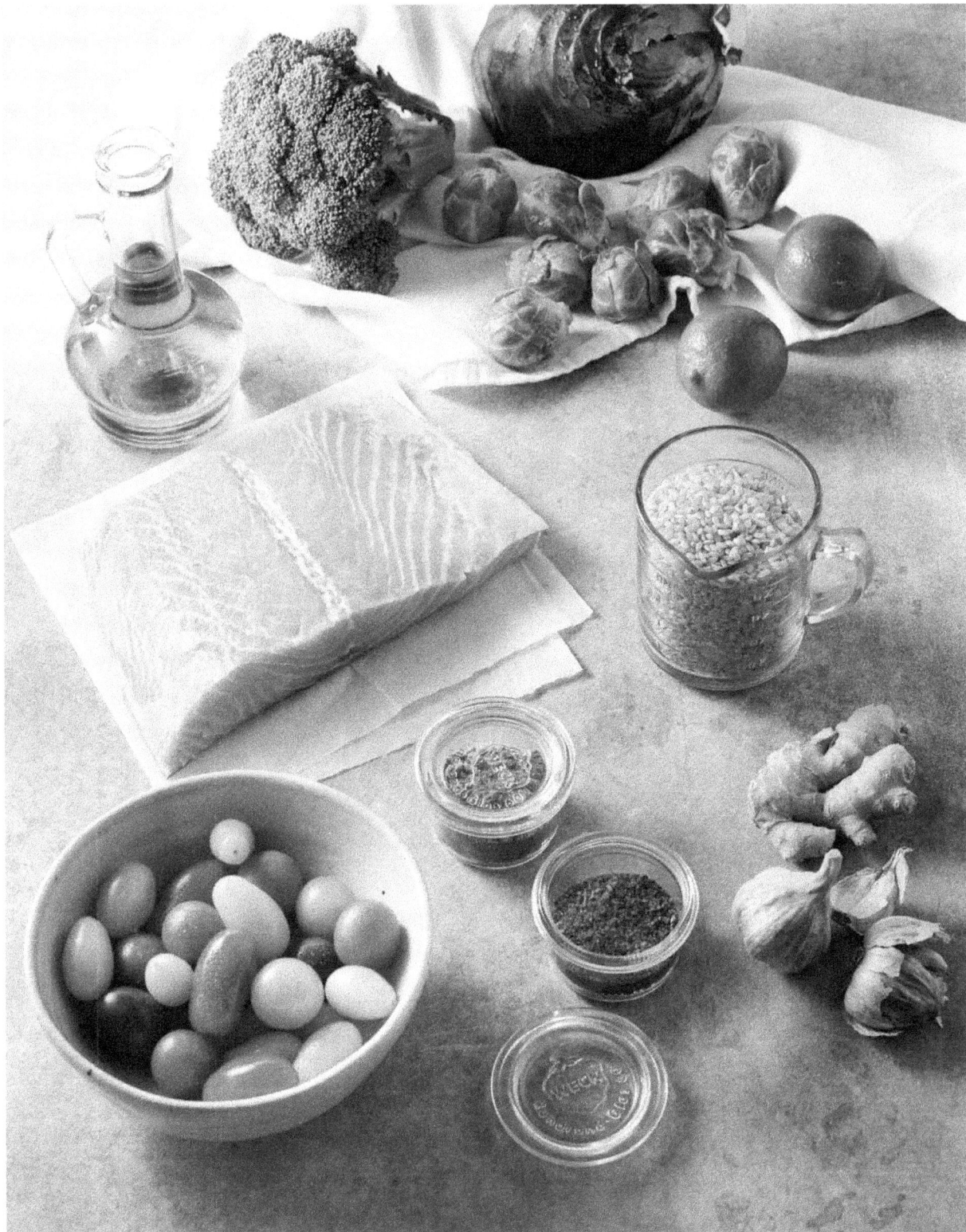

Contents

6 Fish and Seafood

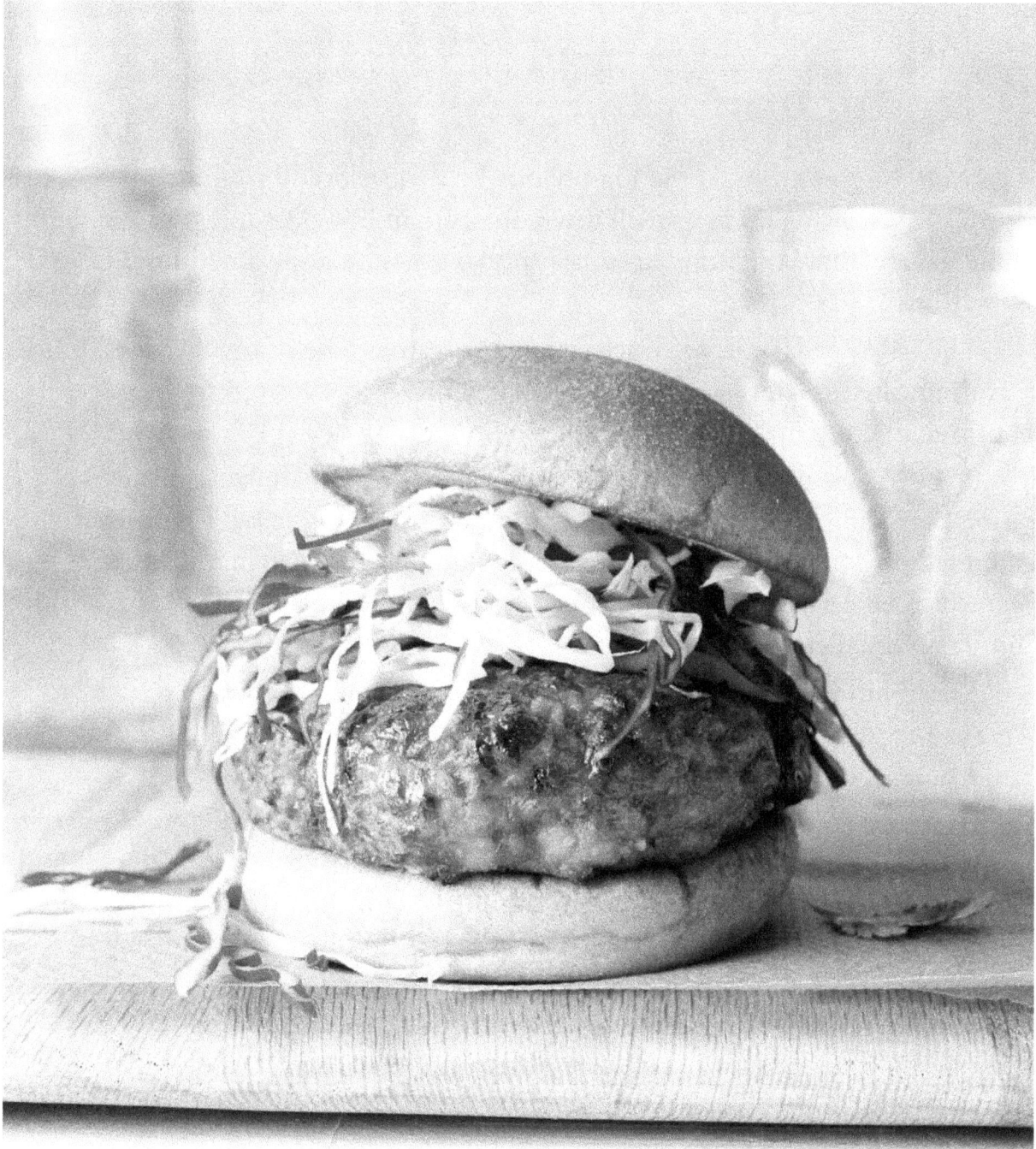

HOISIN TURKEY BURGERS

Introduction

As a teen, I never dreamed the food habits I was developing would come back to haunt me. Growing up in a small town of less than 2,000 people, our restaurant choices were limited. Eating out was a special occasion and something I looked forward to.

The fried foods I ate when we were out became some of my favorites, but it wasn't until years later I realized my eating habits were causing my weight to continue to creep up.

The struggle to maintain a healthier weight has been an issue for me for years. Balancing life as a busy working mother isn't always easy. One area that often fell through the cracks for me was cooking healthy, balanced meals. It seemed to take a lot of time, effort, and energy to meal plan and prepare healthy dinners every night.

I tried different deprivation-themed diets, but I always ended up back at square one. As a registered nurse, I knew that these fad diets weren't the answer and I needed to start more simply.

As I have gotten older my body has changed, and it has become even harder to lose weight and keep it off. I was diagnosed with an autoimmune disease and some of the medications can interfere with my weight-loss efforts. Instead of giving up, I started looking for alternatives that didn't involve completely cutting out certain food groups or food items from my life.

I realized that if I was going to see success, I needed to find ways to make foods I love healthier. The air fryer has been a game changer for me. I can make so many of my favorite recipes significantly healthier, and they taste as good and some are even better than before.

There is a whole new world of opportunities available when it comes to making delicious vegetables that I look forward to eating. Protein is no longer limited to a few boring basics. The air fryer delivers a crispy texture to many of my favorite foods, and there is no guilt involved because only an insignificant amount of olive oil is required.

I am a firm believer that baby steps can change the world. Limiting my fat intake and reducing the calories on many recipes can make a difference on the scale. It also makes a difference inside my body and for my overall health.

This cookbook shows everyday families how to make easy and classic recipes a little bit healthier using the air fryer. This cookbook has recipes for real people. The ingredients are common and can easily be found at any grocery store. I adapted recipes my family has been eating for years, and my family is even more excited to come to the table when they see I am cooking their favorite meals with the air fryer!

I am 100 percent sold on the benefits of air frying. As you begin to use your air fryer, I think you will quickly see how easy it is to adapt regular recipes into healthier versions by cooking them this way. This is an appliance for everyday life, and it deserves space on the counter in your kitchen.

Get ready to learn all about air frying and how it can change how you cook your meals. Keep reading to find recipes that are simple, use just a few ingredients, and don't require you spend the whole evening in the kitchen.

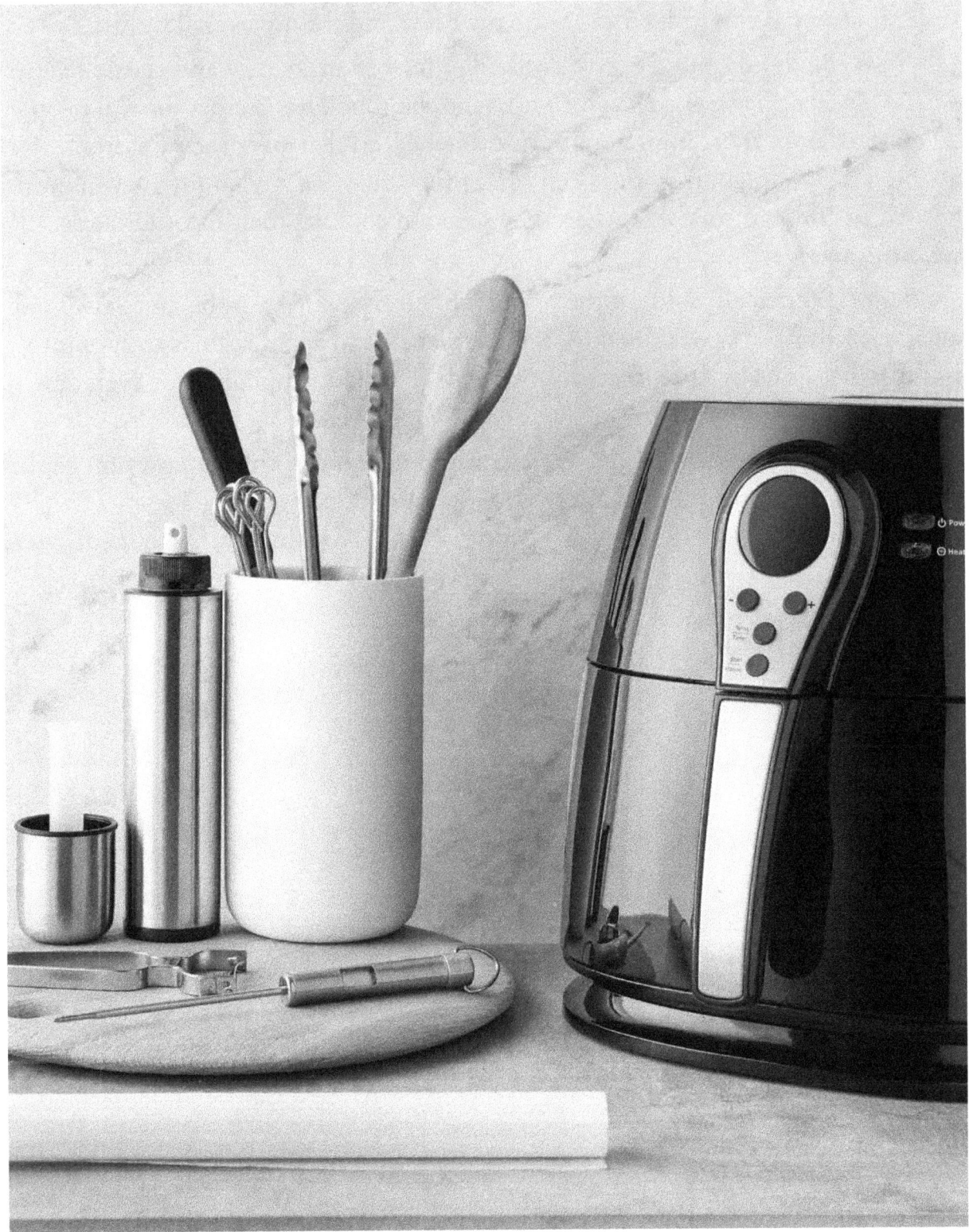

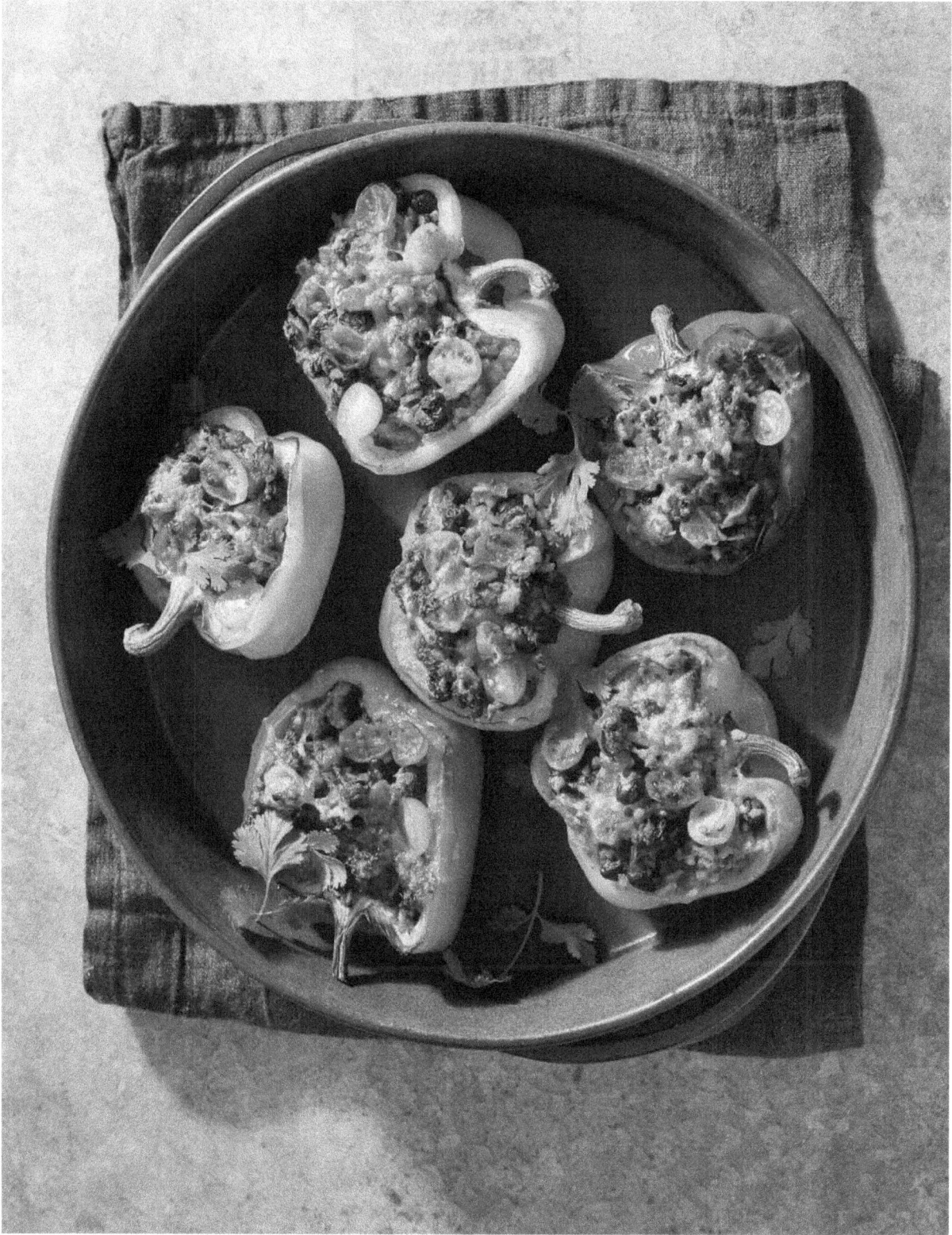

STUFFED BELL PEPPERS

CHAPTER 1

How the Air Fryer Can Help You Lose Weight

Losing weight ultimately comes down to calories. In this chapter, you'll learn how the air fryer is a powerful tool to help you work toward your weight loss goals. It cooks foods using less oil, meaning fewer calories, without sacrificing any of the satisfying flavor and texture you associate with fried foods. Making these kinds of small changes in your diet can have a long-term impact on your overall weight and health.

Although it may be tempting to jump right into this book's delicious air fryer recipes, it's important that you read the first two chapters. Getting to know the air fryer will help make the cooking experience all the more enjoyable.

Why Air Fry?

Weight loss is a personal journey for each person. My struggles to lose weight have helped me realize that wellness isn't only about a number on the scale. There has been a shift in my thinking that has allowed me to see the value of incorporating healthier habits overall into my life and the lives of my family.

Crash diets, on the other hand, don't work for me. Depriving myself of certain foods has never helped me maintain my weight loss goals. If I'm forbidden from eating a food I love for very long, I end up reverting to my old eating habits. A slow-and-steady approach works much better for me, and that means finding ways to cook my favorite foods in healthier ways.

Which leads me to the air fryer. It allows me to enjoy the soul-satisfying flavor and texture of fried foods, without all the calories of traditional frying. It cooks food by circulating hot air around the food very quickly. Typical air fryers have a removable basket that doesn't have to be submerged into hot oil to get foods crispy. Instead, there are holes that let the very hot air move around the food.

Traditionally fried foods are often extremely high in unhealthy fats and very high in calories. It is hard to lose weight if fried foods are on the menu often. But completely eliminating fried foods from our diet can lead us to feel deprived and throws us off our weight-loss goals. Fortunately, French fries do not have to be an off-limits treat if they are made using the air fryer. It is possible to make crunchy homemade fish sticks, chicken strips, and even snacks in the air fryer. The calorie savings will be big, because you'll need much less oil to make these foods in the air fryer.

But it's not just carb-heavy foods that benefit from air frying. One of my favorite things about the air fryer is that it has made vegetables exciting to me again. I have always been a picky eater, and in the past, I wasn't overly eager to try new vegetables. Brussels sprouts were never on my menu until I started cooking them in the air fryer. So, cooking vegetables in the air fryer has been a game changer for me. It is so easy to create delicious and flavorful side dishes using fresh or frozen veggies.

Air frying can be as easy or as complicated as you choose. Start off making simple recipes with common ingredients. Roasted vegetables and shrimp are great choices for beginners. For a simple dish that impresses, you can get the job done with three components: a vegetable, some seasonings, and a little bit of olive oil will give you a scrumptious result.

When you are more comfortable with the appliance try your hand at some more complex recipes. Learning to cook salmon and other seafood recipes will bring healthy proteins and low calories to your plate. Lean cuts of meat turn out moist and delicious in the air fryer.

The more you use the air fryer, the more you will come to value this appliance as a resource in your weight-loss and wellness journey.

Foods to Enjoy

For a well-balanced diet that can still work with your weight loss goals, you'll want to focus on eating high-quality carbohydrates (mostly vegetables), healthy fats, and lean proteins. Fortunately, the air fryer is a great tool for preparing many different foods that fall into these categories.

Veggies

Vegetables are a key component for pretty much any weight loss program. Vegetables are packed with fiber, water, and nutrients, and they tend to be lower in calories than other foods. They're also a good source of healthy carbohydrates (more on that shortly).

The problem is that when we are trying to eat only healthy foods, vegetable boredom can hit quickly. We get stuck in a rut eating the same few choice all the time. Suddenly we find ourselves snacking on a bag of chips instead of carrot sticks.

Finding delicious new ways to prepare vegetables is imperative for long term weight loss. Air-fried veggies can have a roasted taste with a slightly crispy texture. These results are achieved without a lot of unnecessary oil. I love the flexibility of being able to air fry fresh vegetables with no pre-cooking required. Spicy Sweet Potatoes and Simple Roasted Cauliflower are on our menu almost every week.

Healthy Fats

Fats in general have a bad reputation. It's true that we want to avoid consuming trans fats and saturated fats, especially when trying to lose weight. But there are also healthy fats, which are critical for us to produce energy, support cell growth, absorb certain nutrients, and produce certain hormones.

Monounsaturated and polyunsaturated fats are considered good fats. Some common foods that are high in good fats include avocados, nuts, seeds, and fish. There are also specific oils that are lower in saturated fat thus making them a better choice. The oils lowest in saturated fats are avocado, canola, corn, olive, grapeseed, safflower, peanut, sesame, soybean, and sunflower.

When I am preparing foods in the air fryer and oil is needed, I typically use an olive oil spray. Very little oil is required for air frying. Lightly spraying foods with a spritz of olive oil can add that crunchy texture we crave from fried foods, but without all the calories that traditional deep-frying would add.

Lean Proteins

Protein helps you feel full longer, and if you aren't hungry, you won't be tempted to snack or eat as much during your next meal. An additional benefit of protein is the help it gives your body in maintaining lean muscle mass.

However, not all protein is created equal. Some sources of protein like fatty cuts of meat, hot dogs, bacon, and other processed meats are very high in saturated fat. It's important to choose lean proteins if you are trying to lose weight. Opt for turkey, chicken, and lean cuts of beef and pork when planning your meals. Easy Turkey Tenderloin, Whole Roasted Chicken, and Lemon-Garlic Tilapia are just a few of the protein-packed recipes in this cookbook.

Protein is known to reduce the hunger hormone ghrelin and boost levels of the peptide YY, which makes you feel full.

High-Quality Carbohydrates

Potatoes and sweet potatoes seem to be controversial vegetables when it comes to weight loss. Both of these potatoes are highly nutritious. They are rich in fiber and vitamins B_6 and C. There is a difference of where these potatoes fall on the glycemic index. Sweet potatoes have a lower glycemic index than regular white potatoes. Potatoes have a lot to offer and can help you feel full faster. The key is to pair them with lean protein and avoid slathering them with butter or other high-fat condiments.

In addition to vegetables, other high-quality carbohydrates include foods like beans and other legumes, fruits, and whole grains. In addition to being packed with nutrients and minerals, they also help limit fluctuations in our insulin levels and regulate our blood sugar.

It is common to feel hungry and overeat after a blood-sugar spike. Low-quality carbohydrates such as processed foods, white bread, desserts, juices, and other sugary drinks can cause these spikes to occur. It is very difficult to lose weight eating a diet high in low-quality carbohydrates.

I have discovered delicious swaps for highly processed carbs, and I don't feel at all deprived. Swapping out spaghetti noodles for zucchini noodles or using riced cauliflower in place of white rice are two easy replacements. The air fryer is a tool I use to turn plain high-quality carbohydrates into tasty dishes my whole family loves. The best part is that I am cooking with whole foods packed with nutrients my body needs.

Keep reading to learn how combining air frying with simple spices from the pantry can turn high-quality carbs into flavorful, healthy side dishes and snacks.

Foods to Avoid

There are certain foods and ingredients that should be avoided when you're trying to lose weight. The recipes in the books don't include these ingredients, but you'll find the air fryer is particularly good at producing satisfying results without them.

As mentioned previously, trans fat does nothing to enhance your body or your health. It raises the bad cholesterol level (LDL) and lowers the good cholesterol level (HDL) in our body. Trans fats have been shown to increase our risk of heart disease, stroke, and even type 2 diabetes. Trans fats tend to be found in processed foods and will be listed on packages as "partially hydrogenated oils" in the ingredient list. Common processed foods that are high in trans fat include crackers, chips, cookies, cakes, fast food, and vegetable shortening. There can be some hidden sources of trans fat in items like coffee creamer and baked goods.

Though many of us have a sweet tooth, sugar definitely goes on the forbidden list. And it lurks in many processed foods like salad dressings, pasta sauces, bread, canned fruit, and even in foods labeled as diet foods. Sugar adds calories without filling us up and can even lead to food cravings.

High-carb snacks are a common pitfall when dieting. Chips, crackers, granola bars, and other highly processed foods fall into this category. They contain "empty" calories with little-to-no nutritional value for our bodies.

While low-fat foods may sound like a good option, unless they are a naturally low-fat whole food, it's best to avoid these items. They may be lower in fat, but it's usually replaced by sugar. Additionally, these foods are generally not as flavorful, and people tend to overeat them.

Fruit juice is not a healthy option. It is high in calories, which aren't very filling or satisfying when consumed in liquid form. The fiber from the fruit, which helps you to feel full, has been stripped away. Eating whole fruit is a much better choice.

The Plate Approach to Weight Loss

You may feel a little overwhelmed by the dos and don'ts we just covered when it comes to making smart food choices for weight loss. But don't worry, there's one area in which we are going to make things simple: This cookbook is not going to take a calorie-counting approach to weight loss. Instead, I want to focus on a simpler way to think about mealtime: the plate approach.

The plate approach focuses our attention on what's in front of us at mealtime and divides it up into sections. Half of our plate should be filled with vegetables. The other half of the plate should be filled with healthy fats, lean proteins, and high-quality carbohydrates. What I love about the plate approach is that it doesn't require a membership, calorie-counting, or even food tracking. It's a way of eating that anyone can do, and you can start immediately.

Keep in mind portion control when you are filling your plate. Using a smaller plate will help you keep your portions in control and also tricks your brain into thinking your plate is fuller.

A sectioned portion-control plate makes a wonderful tool to help you get used to the plate approach. But you can you also use something as easy as your own two hands to provide an easy visual reminder about portion sizes. Women should eat a palm-sized piece of lean protein plus a fistful of veggies at each meal. Add 25 percent more of each of those if you're a man. As for the rest of your plate, no one should have more than a cupped handful of high-quality carbs or a thumb's worth of healthy fats per meal.

This cookbook will make it easy for you to use the recipes to fill your plate appropriately. You won't have to take the time to count calories or input ingredients into a food tracker with the simple plate approach to dieting. All you need to do is fill your plate with healthy portion sizes of vegetables and other high-quality carbs, lean proteins, and healthy fats.

IF YOU'RE COUNTING CALORIES

Each person must decide the best approach to weight loss for themselves. For some, that means counting calories.

There are about 3,500 calories in one pound of stored body fat. If you can subtract 3,500 calories from your intake through diet and/or exercise you will lose one pound of body weight.

Experts say that the average person requires about 2,000 calories a day to maintain their current weight. This number will vary based on your height, weight, age, gender, and your current level of physical activity.

An easy way to begin counting calories is to use a food tracking app or website. It will help you calculate your basal metabolic rate (BMR), which is the amount of energy (calories) your body needs while resting. Knowing your BMR will help you set a daily calorie goal.

This cookbook contains calories counts for every recipe. There are also occasional tips on how to make a recipe even lower in calories.

My 10 Tips for Success

Whether you're using the plate method or following a diet that requires more specific tracking, there are some universal best practices that will help make your weight-loss goals a reality. Here are 10 tips to follow if you want to see a positive change on the scale.

1. **Don't drink your calories.** Stick to drinking water as much as

possible. If you prefer flavored drinks, try adding some fruit slices to your water. Tea is another good option if you don't load it with sugar.

2. **Get enough sleep each night.** More and more research shows how sleep deprivation can lead to weight gain. Quality sleep is vital to good health and helps give us the energy to stay active during the day.

3. **Plan your meals out each week.** Even if you're not counting calories, meal planning can help you avoid spur of the moment trips through the fast-food drive-through. Be sure to account for breakfast, lunch, dinner, and snacks.

4. **Prep your food.** You'll start your week off right by prepping all your snacks for the week. Portion out food into baggies and containers so you can grab it and go. For snacks, wash and cut up vegetables and fruits so they are ready to eat. Mornings are a breeze if your lunches are prepped and ready to go the night before.

5. **Stock up on healthy foods.** It's hard to make healthy choices if your home is full of processed and unhealthy foods. Clear your refrigerator and pantry of these culprits and stock up on healthier alternatives.

6. **Keep moving.** Staying active is an important part of any weight loss plan, so find ways to exercise that you enjoy. Try to change your exercise routine from time to time so your body doesn't hit a plateau. Fitness trackers are an easy way to spot check how much you're moving throughout the day.

7. **Purchase a smaller plate.** There are special divided plates that are designed for weight loss, or you can get a child's plate. Just remember to always fill the largest section with vegetables at each meal.

8. **Variety makes a difference.** Eating the same thing all the time gets boring fast. Keep your diet varied and try new recipes and new foods each week. I like to keep a binder in the kitchen that's packed with healthy recipes and weight loss tips.

9. **Visual reminders are helpful.** I have found it useful to keep a picture of myself at a healthy weight in the kitchen. I see this picture when I open the refrigerator, and it helps me keep my food choices in

perspective with my goals. If you are working to lose weight before a big vacation or event, it may help to hang a picture of that location as a reminder.

10. **Positive affirmations are extremely motivating.** What we say to ourselves can have a huge impact on our ability to find success with weight loss. Speak kindly to yourself and remain positive. I like to hang positive messages on the refrigerator to remind myself that I am worth the effort!

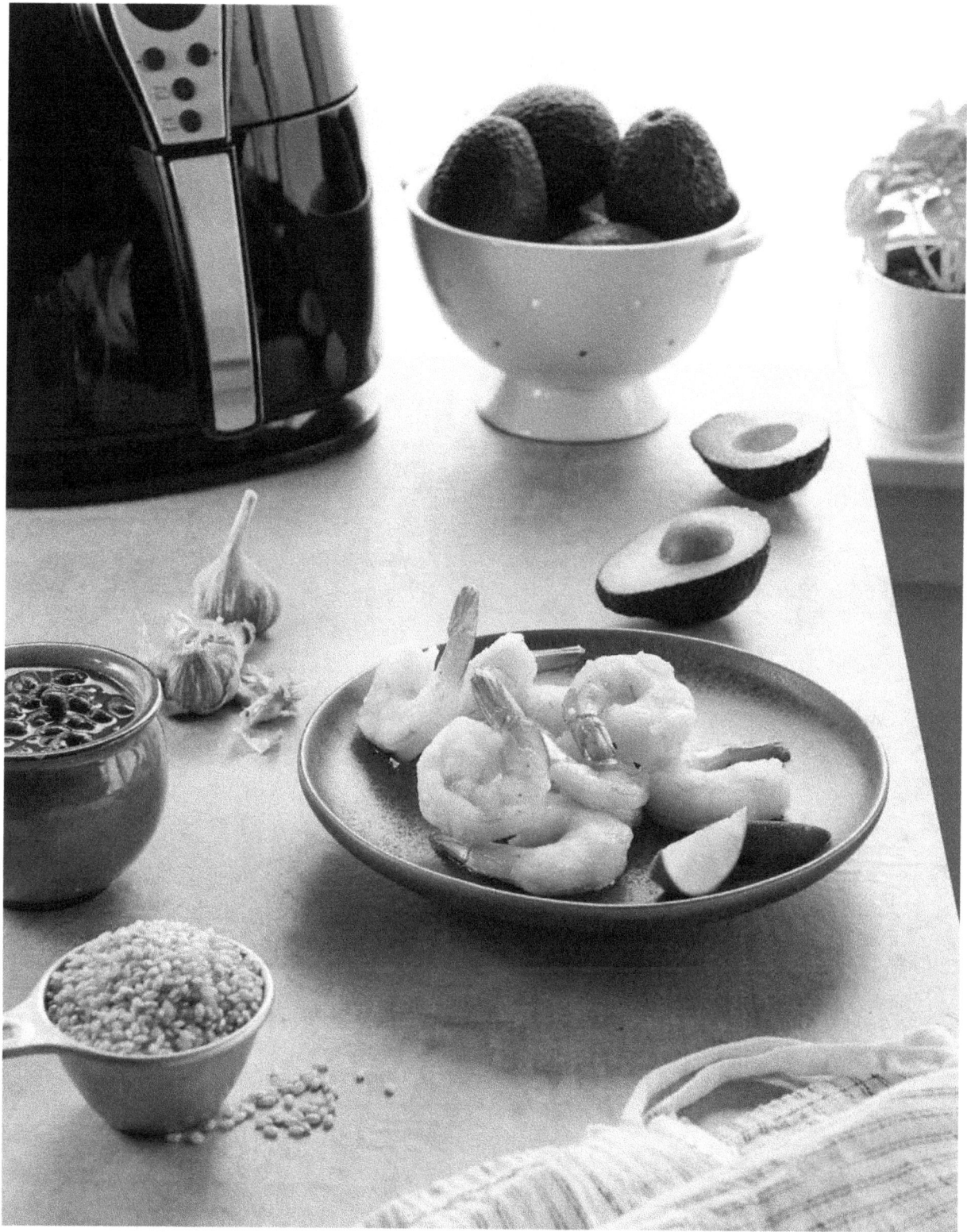

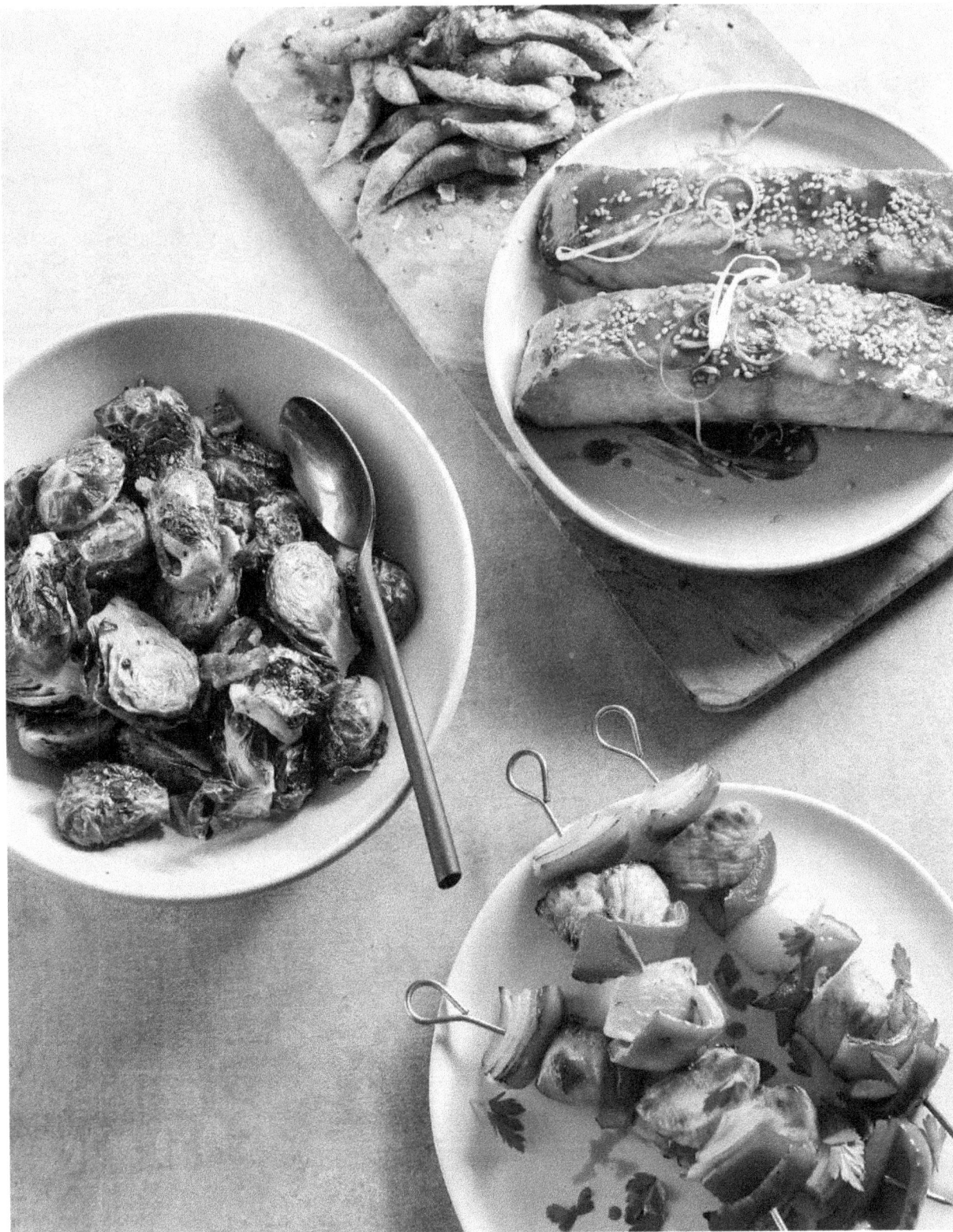

GARLIC EDAMAME
SESAME-GLAZED SALMON
BACON ROASTED BRUSSELS SPROUTS
HAWAIIAN PINEAPPLE CHICKEN KEBABS

CHAPTER 2

Fire Up the Air Fryer

One of the best things about the air fryer is how simple it is to use. Getting to know your air fryer will give you the confidence to start cooking your favorite foods with less oil and fewer calories. This chapter provides tips, tools, and troubleshooting advice that will allow you to get healthy meals on the table right away. You'll also learn to set up your kitchen in a way that will make it easy to stick to your goals. Finally, this chapter provides a meal plan to make starting your weight-loss journey as easy as possible.

My Kitchen Secrets

There are certain foods and accessories that will allow you to take full advantage of what the air fryer has to offer. Follow these guidelines to get your kitchen and pantry prepped and ready to start making healthy meals.

Healthy Air Fryer Staples

You will see some ingredients used over and over throughout this cookbook's recipes. To set yourself up for success, stock your refrigerator and pantry with these heathy air-fryer staples.

Boneless, Skinless Chicken Breasts: This protein is versatile and can be used in many different recipes. You can make quick lunches and dinners with boneless, skinless chicken breasts, and you'll be surprised by how tasty chicken can be in the air fryer.

Chickpeas: A high-fiber, high-protein snack, chickpeas only take minutes to cook in the air fryer and can be seasoned lots of different ways.

Eggs: An easy-to-get, inexpensive source of protein, eggs are surprisingly delicious in the air fryer and can be used in a variety of dishes.

Extra-Virgin Olive Oil: Olive oil is a must-have for air frying. There's a myth that no oil is needed when using an air fryer. Using small amounts of extra-virgin olive oil or avocado oil will give you that fried taste without the calories that come from deep-fat frying. Extra-virgin olive oil and avocado oil are both healthy fats and play an important part of any healthy diet. When I call for "olive oil" in the recipes, I always mean "extra-virgin olive oil."

Fresh Vegetables: As previously mentioned, veggies rise to delicious new heights when air-fried. Keep vegetables like sweet potatoes, broccoli, and cauliflower on hand for simple and delicious side dishes or snacks.

Lean Ground Turkey: A tasty lower-fat alternative to ground beef, lean ground turkey is a versatile protein. It can easily be made into meatballs or burgers in the air fryer.

Shrimp: Extremely easy to cook in the air fryer, shrimp can be made with a variety of seasonings and sauces and the outcome is always delicious. I like to keep bags of frozen shrimp in the freezer all the time for fast, simple meals.

Whole Grains: Keep whole grains like quinoa or brown rice in the pantry to round out your meal. Or use them as base to turn veggies and protein into a full meal in a bowl.

Whole-Wheat Panko Bread Crumbs: Use bread crumbs to transform everyday dishes into a crunchy, addictive experience. They can be seasoned a variety of ways to change the flavor of a dish.

Spice Up Your Life

Spices can brighten up the flavor of otherwise boring ingredients and can be mixed and matched to add variety to your dining routine. You'll be more satisfied with your meals and less inclined to overeat.

All-Purpose Seasoning Salt: I love the convenience of salt blends. The combination of salt and other spices tastes great on almost any protein or vegetable.

Black Pepper: This universal spice adds subtle heat to dishes and also offers digestive health benefits.

Cajun Seasoning: My personal favorite spice blend, this lively, brightly flavored combination of spices such as paprika, cayenne pepper, chili flakes, and more can bring a vibrant kick to any dish.

Cayenne Pepper: It only takes a tiny amount of cayenne to bring a delightful heat to a recipe. It has also been said to boost metabolism and curb hunger.

Cinnamon: One of the healthiest spices, cinnamon brings a depth of flavor to sweet and savory dishes. Two big benefits of cinnamon are the ability to help lower blood sugar levels and to reduce heart disease risk factors.

Cumin: With its aromatic, nutty flavor, cumin is a staple in many spice blends. It also helps aid digestion and is a source of iron.

Garlic Powder: Made from dehydrated, ground garlic cloves, garlic powder has anti-inflammatory qualities and adds a homey flavor to many recipes.

Onion Powder: Get the flavor of onion without the hassle of teary eyes. Onion powder is made of dehydrated, ground onions. It contains the helpful mineral magnesium which can aid in the production of energy.

Paprika: Use this spice to add a wonderful peppery, smoky flavor to foods. Since it's made from ground bell peppers, it's loaded with vitamins, minerals, and antioxidants.

Salt: A mainstay of pretty much every recipe, salt can help bring out new flavors in foods. The essential minerals of sodium and chloride in salt act as important electrolytes in the body. These minerals are essential for fluid balance, nerve transmission, and muscle function. There are several kinds of salt to keep on hand: table salt, kosher salt, and sea salt.

Seafood Seasoning: You can make an amazing air-fried seafood dish with basic seafood seasoning. This seasoning will save you time and add a lot of flavor to your fish. Seafood seasonings usually contain a mixture of allspice, celery seed, salt, mustard powder, pepper, paprika, and more.

MUST-HAVE TOOLS

While using the air fryer is as simple as can be, there are some helpful tools and accessories that will make preparing the healthy recipes in this book even easier.

Baking Pan: A baking pan that will fit inside the fryer basket opens a whole new realm of recipe possibilities. It allows you to cook foods in the air fryer that you would traditionally cook in the oven. Frittatas and casseroles can be cooked in a baking pan in the air fryer.

Cooking Rack with Skewers: When cooking meat and vegetable kebobs, the raised rack allows total air circulation around the food, so you get a wonderful, crispy result.

Heat-Resistant Tongs: Tongs are used to turn food during cooking and remove it from the fryer basket. It is important to have tongs that have silicone tips, so they don't scratch the fryer basket.

Meat Thermometer: Cooking meat to the proper internal temperature is important to avoid food-borne illnesses, and it also takes any guesswork out of knowing when the meat is done.

Oil Spray Bottle: You can buy many different types of misters and spray bottles that allow you to spray a light coating of olive oil or avocado oil on foods and into the fryer basket. Just make sure whatever you buy is non-aerosol.

Parchment Liners: Liners help keep food from sticking to the fryer basket. These are extremely helpful when preparing seafood. Air fryer–specific liners work best because they have holes that allow the air to continue to circulate around the food despite the liner.

Step-by-Step Air Frying

The ease of using an air fryer is one of the things that makes it an invaluable tool in your weight-loss repertoire. Follow these simple steps, and you'll be an air-frying expert in no time.

1. Always read the manual that comes with your air fryer before using it. Each air fryer brand has slightly different guidelines and suggestions that will help make your air-frying experience better.

2. It is important to wash the basket and crisper plate (if your unit has one) before using it the first time. Use hot, soapy water to wash, rinse, and dry the basket. Do not use abrasive cleaners, steel wool, or scouring pads to clean the fryer basket.

3. Be sure the air intake vent and/or air outlet vents are not blocked while the air fryer is in use. This could cause the unit to overheat.

4. Check your owner's manual to see if your air fryer needs to be preheated before use. Some models recommend a few minutes of preheat time, and others do not require any preheating.

5. When a recipe requires that you cut up the food, make sure to create similar-sized pieces so the food cooks evenly in the air fryer, and always put food in an even, single layer in the fryer basket for the best results.

6. Set the timer and the temperature setting on the air fryer and press start.

7. Check periodically to make sure you're not overcooking, at least when you first make a recipe. You can also open the drawer to shake, toss, or turn food over during cooking. The recipes in this book will let you know when this is required.

8. Remember that the fryer basket will be extremely hot during and after use. Always use oven mitts or hot pads when handling the basket.

9. When finished, do not overturn the air fryer unit to get food out of the basket. Remove the basket from the unit or use heat-safe tongs to remove food from inside the basket.

CLEANING THE AIR FRYER

Before you start your air-frying adventure, it is important to clean the air fryer properly.

Remove any Packaging and Tape. Start off by removing any packaging materials from inside the unit and taking any tape off the unit.

Wash the Basket. Wash the fryer basket in hot, soapy water. If your unit has a removable crisper plate, this also needs to be washed in hot, soapy water. Rinse the items off and dry them thoroughly.

Dishwasher Safety. There are many different brands and styles of air fryers on the market. Always check your owner's guide to find out if your fryer basket is dishwasher safe before washing it in the dishwasher.

Food Residue. If your fryer basket has difficult food residue stuck inside, soak the basket in a sink filled with warm, soapy water.

Heating Element. If the heating element of your air fryer gets dirty and has food particles on it, the best way to clean it is to use a small cleaning brush to remove the food residue.

Main Unit. You cannot soak or immerse the main air fryer unit in water! Keep the unit clean by wiping it down with a damp cloth. Remember to always unplug the unit before wiping it down.

Perfect Air Frying, Every Time

While using the air fryer couldn't be simpler, there are a few tricks and tips to take your fry skills to the next level.

Watch the food. It's important to keep an eye on your food while it cooks, especially when you are first starting out. Food will cook at different speeds depending on the size of your fryer.

Shake the basket. Shaking the fryer basket can really improve the outcome of your food. If you're cooking smaller items like chopped vegetables, French fries, etc., be sure to pause the cooking a few times and shake the basket a little bit. This will help the food get crunchy all the way around and not stick to the basket.

Oil adds crunch. You still need to use a little bit of oil in an air fryer. It doesn't take very much oil to achieve a crunchy result. Spray the fryer basket lightly with olive oil before adding your ingredients to prevent food from sticking to the basket. It is also helpful to spray the food lightly with olive oil to get a crispier texture. The recipes will indicate if this step is necessary.

Use a meat thermometer. Check your meat for doneness with a meat thermometer. This will help you get perfectly cooked meat.

Recipe conversion is easy. It is easy to convert recipes from your conventional oven. Just reduce the temperature of the air fryer by 25°F. Check on the food periodically to avoid overcooking.

Remove the food from the basket. When the food is done cooking, remove it from the fryer basket immediately to prevent the food from becoming overcooked.

Secure lightweight foods. When cooking lightweight food, the circulating air may blow the foods around in the basket. You can alleviate this issue by securing foods with toothpicks or even a pie weight.

Cooking time depends on food size. Smaller ingredients will typically require a shorter cooking time than larger ones.

Troubleshooting

There are some common problems you may encounter when using your air fryer. Read through these troubleshooting tips so you are ready if any issues arise.

My food is burnt. It is very easy to overcook food in an air fryer until you get the hang of it. My best advice is to watch the food very closely for doneness. It is not a problem to open the air fryer and look in the basket a few times throughout cooking.

Food is sticking to the fryer basket. Mist your basket with olive oil before adding ingredients. This will help prevent food from sticking to the basket. You can also use fryer basket parchment liners.

The air fryer is smoking. The most common cause for smoking is if you are cooking foods that are naturally high in fat. Some of the excess fat may be in the bottom of the air fryer during the cooking process. You can reduce the likelihood of smoke by draining the fat out of the bottom of the air fryer part way through the cooking time. Another tip is to put a tablespoon or two of water under the basket. This will reduce any smoke during the cooking process.

My food does not seem crispy. The best way to ensure the food you air fry comes out crispy is to lightly mist the food with olive oil before cooking. Certain foods and recipes can benefit from a light mist of olive oil midway through the cooking time to add the best crunch to the recipe.

My fryer basket is sticky or flaking. If you are using aerosol cooking sprays, they can cause problems with the fryer basket over time. These non-stick cooking sprays can damage the basket. Remember to always use non-aerosol oils for your air fryer.

My air fryer smells like burnt plastic. Some people report that their air fryer has a burnt plastic smell when they first start using it. Typically, this smell will go away after the first few uses. If the smell continues after that, I would advise contacting the manufacturer for a recommendation.

Fry Time: Healthy Foods

One of my favorite parts of air frying is the ease of cooking healthy foods. This fry time table will give you a cheat sheet to refer to when you are experimenting with your favorite healthy foods. The recipes in this cookbook may have different variations from this chart, but the chart is a good jumping off point when you are starting your air fryer journey.

Fresh Food	Quantity	Time	Temperature	Notes
Apple chips	2 apples	8 to 12 mins	350°F	Sliced thin, shake basket
Asparagus	1 bunch	8 to 12 mins	390°F	Trim ends
Broccoli	1 head	10 to 12 mins	390°F	Cut in 1-inch florets
Broccoli, frozen	1 pound	20 mins	390°F	Shake every 5 minutes
Brussels sprouts	1 pound	15 to 20 mins	390°F	Cut in half, stem removed
Carrots	1 pound	13 to 16 mins	390°F	Cut in ½-inch slices
Cauliflower	1 head	15 to 20 mins	390°F	Cut in 1-inch florets
Chickpeas	15 ounces	15 to 20 mins	390°F	Shake every 5 minutes
Corn on the cob	2 ears	6 to 10 mins	360°F	Whole, husks removed
Corn, frozen	2 ears	15 to 18 mins	360°F	
Edamame	2 cups	10 to 15 mins	390°F	Whole, shake halfway
Green beans, fresh	12 ounces	8 to 10 mins	390°F	Trim ends
Green beans, frozen	12 ounces	18 to 20 mins	390°F	Shake every 5 minutes
Mixed vegetables	1 pound	15 to 20 mins	400°F	Cut into ½-inch chunks
Mushrooms	8 ounces	5 to 7 mins	400°F	Cut in 1-inch pieces
Okra, fresh	1 pound	8 to 12 mins	350°F	Cut into ½-inch slices
Okra, frozen	1 pound	20 mins	350°F	Shake every 5 minutes
Potatoes, baby	1 pound	15 to 17 mins	400°F	Whole
Potatoes, russet	1 pound	18 to 20 mins	390°F	Cut in 1-inch wedges

Potatoes, sweet	1 pound	15 to 20 mins	390°F	Cut in 1-inch chunks
Squash	1 pound	12 to 15 mins	400°F	Cut in 1-inch chunks
Zucchini	1 pound	12 to 15 mins	400°F	Cut in 1-inch sticks
Chicken breasts	2 breasts	18 to 22 mins	375°F	Use boneless
Chicken drumsticks	1 pound	18 to 22 mins	370°F	Don't crowd in basket
Chicken tenders	1 pound	8 to 12 mins	360°F	Fresh, hand-breaded
Pork chops	1 pound	13 to 16 mins	375°F	Boneless
Pork tenderloin	1 pound	20 to 25 mins	370°F	Whole
Burger	4 (4-oz) patties	8 to 10 mins	375°F	Lean ground beef or turkey
Meatballs	1 pound	5 to 8 mins	375°F	1-inch meatballs
Rib eye steak	2 (8-oz) steaks	10 to 15 mins	400°F	Bone-in
Sirloin steak	2 (8-oz) steaks	10 to 20 mins	390°F	Whole
Calamari	1 pound	4 to 8 mins	400°F	Cut into rings, hand-breaded
Fish fillets	4 (8-oz) fillets	10 to 12 mins	400°F	Fresh, hand-breaded
Salmon fillets	2 (4-oz) fillets	10 to 13 mins	390°F	Brushed with oil
Scallops	1 pound	5 to 7 mins	400°F	Shake basket during cooking
Shrimp, fresh	1 pound	7 to 10 mins	390°F	Peeled, tails on, tossed in oil
Shrimp, frozen	1 pound	10 to 12 mins	390°F	Peeled, tails on, tossed in oil

About the Recipes

This cookbook includes some of my favorite recipes. I have had so much fun adapting our family recipes for the air fryer. It is like eating these dishes for the very first time. The book includes a large mix of main dishes and side dishes that can be paired together for a delicious meal. Mix and match these recipes so you never get bored at dinner time. You will even find some recipes that are full meals all on their own. You will be amazed at how many foods can be prepared in the air fryer. The cookbook includes recipes for breakfast, healthy snacks, vegetables and side dishes, fish and seafood, poultry, and beef and pork. There is something for everyone! I have tried to include family-friendly recipes to please even the pickiest eaters.

As you browse through the recipes, you'll see that most of the recipes have 10 or fewer ingredients. The ingredients are all commonly available at any grocery store. Making healthy food doesn't have to be overly complicated or expensive.

As you are reading through these recipes be sure to keep an eye out for the recipe labels and tips. Recipes will be labeled if they are dairy-free, gluten-free, or vegetarian. This will help you quickly pick out recipes for different dietary needs. You'll also find tips showing you how to vary recipes to meet those needs, how to make some dishes even lower in calories,what to pair foods with, and how to take your air frying to the next level.

My Favorite Meals for Your First Week

A great way to get comfortable using the air fryer to make the recipes in this book is to start with the tasty suggestions below. These are some of my favorite recipes, and my family loves them, too! I've also included information about how much healthier these air-fried versions are.

Meal	Total Time	Total Calories	Total Fat	How Much Healthier
Breakfast Potatoes	30 minutes	199	1g	Traditional fried breakfast potatoes use 2 tablespoons or more of oil. This recipe only uses 1½ teaspoons of oil! That saves almost 200 calories.
Crunchy Tex-Mex Tortilla Chips	10 minutes	116	2g	Store-bought corn tortilla chips have around 6 grams of fat per serving. Making your own chips in the air fryer will reduce the fat by 4 to 5 grams per serving.
Seafood Spring Rolls and **Sweet**		159	1g	Spring rolls are usually fried in 2 to 3 tablespoons of hot oil. This recipe only

Recipe	Time	Calories	Fat	Notes
and Spicy Broccoli	1 hour	54	1g	uses a misting of olive oil, saving over 200 calories.
Steak Fingers and **Green Beans and New Potatoes**	1 hour	288 / 152	12g / 1g	Fried steak fingers are cooked in hot oil. Air-fried steak fingers are lightly sprayed with oil, saving calories and fat.
Mexican Sheet Pan Dinner	25 minutes	178	6g	Sheet pan dinners typically use 3 tablespoons of oil compared to only a spritzing of oil in this recipe. This can save over 40 grams of fat.

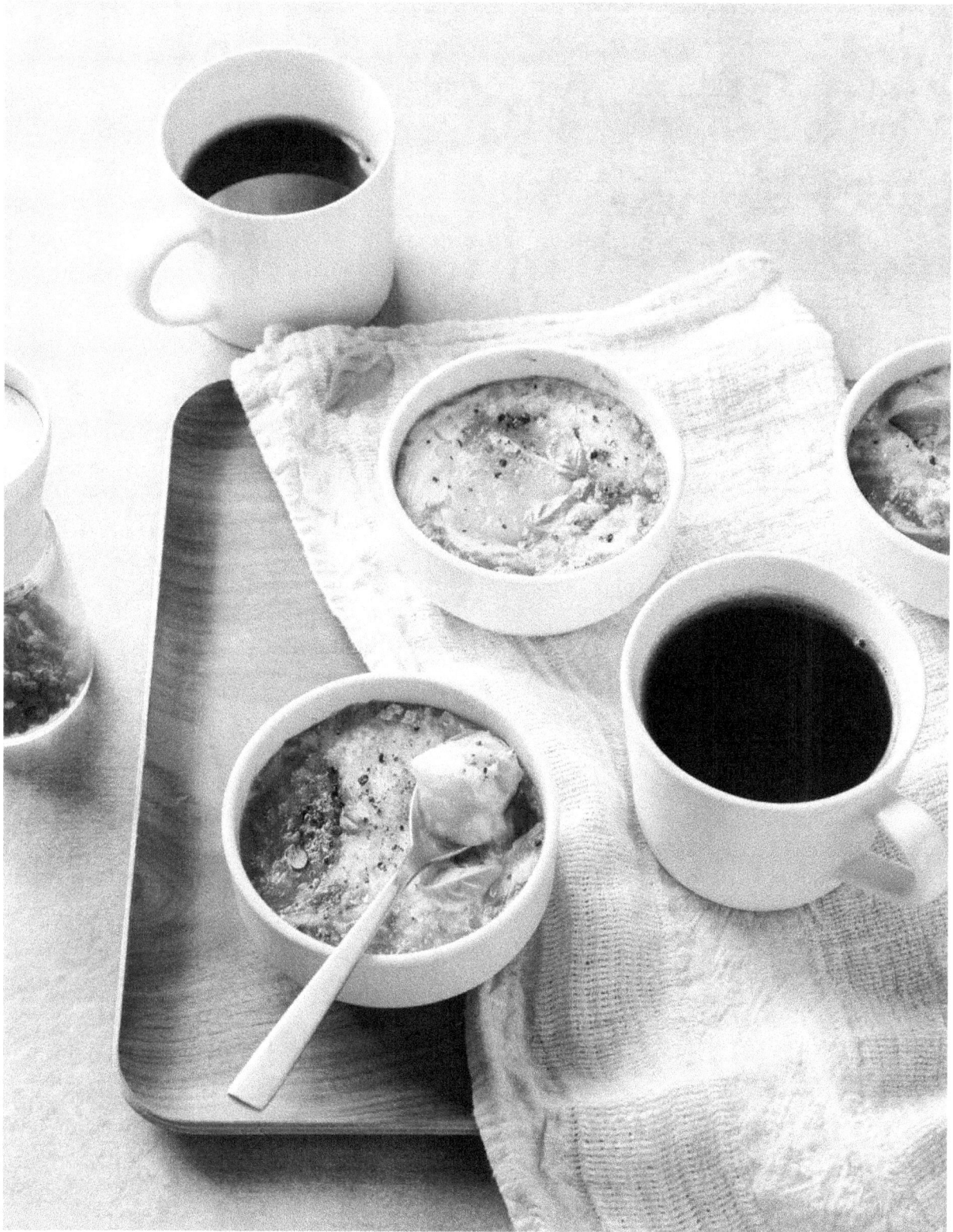

ITALIAN EGG CUPS

Breakfast

Breakfast Potatoes

PREP TIME: 10 MINUTES / **COOK TIME:** 20 MINUTES / **SERVES** 6 / 400°F

Pan-fried potatoes are a breakfast classic, but they're usually saturated with oil. Fortunately, you can get them just as crispy in this guilt-free version. Pair with a poached egg and a piece of turkey sausage for a complete breakfast.

DAIRY-FREE

GLUTEN-FREE

VEGETARIAN

1½ teaspoons olive oil, divided, plus more for misting
4 large potatoes, skins on, cut into cubes
2 teaspoons seasoned salt, divided
1 teaspoon minced garlic, divided
2 large green or red bell peppers, cut into 1-inch chunks
½ onion, diced

1. Lightly mist the fryer basket with olive oil.

2. In a medium bowl, toss the potatoes with ½ teaspoon of olive oil. Sprinkle with 1 teaspoon of seasoned salt and ½ teaspoon of minced garlic. Stir to coat.

3. Place the seasoned potatoes in the fryer basket in a single layer.

4. Cook for 5 minutes. Shake the basket and cook for another 5 minutes.

5. Meanwhile, in a medium bowl, toss the bell peppers and onion with the remaining ½ teaspoon of olive oil.

6. Sprinkle the peppers and onions with the remaining 1 teaspoon of seasoned salt and ½ teaspoon of minced garlic. Stir to coat.

7. Add the seasoned peppers and onions to the fryer basket with the potatoes.

8. Cook for 5 minutes. Shake the basket and cook for an additional 5 minutes.

Air Fry Like a Pro: If you like your breakfast potatoes extra crispy, spray them with a little extra olive oil midway and add a few minutes to the cooking time. However, that will add calories, so be aware.

Per Serving

Calories: 199; Total Fat: 1g; Saturated Fat: <1g; Cholesterol: 0mg; Carbohydrates: 43g; Protein: 5g; Fiber: 7g; Sodium: 507mg

Baked Potato Breakfast Boats

PREP TIME: 10 MINUTES / **COOK TIME:** 20 MINUTES / **SERVES** 4 / 350°F

Need a hand-held breakfast for busy mornings on the go? Crispy potato skins are full of eggs and bacon with a sprinkling of cheese and easy to grab as you run out the door. These are so tasty and filling you can eat them for any meal, and they even make great party snacks.

GLUTEN-FREE

2 large russet potatoes, scrubbed
Olive oil
Salt
Freshly ground black pepper
4 eggs
2 tablespoons chopped, cooked bacon
1 cup shredded cheddar cheese

1. Poke holes in the potatoes with a fork and microwave on full power for 5 minutes.

2. Turn potatoes over and cook an additional 3 to 5 minutes, or until the potatoes are fork tender.

3. Cut the potatoes in half lengthwise and use a spoon to scoop out the inside of the potato. Be careful to leave a layer of potato so that it makes a sturdy "boat."

4. Lightly spray the fryer basket with olive oil. Spray the skin side of the potatoes with oil and sprinkle with salt and pepper to taste.

5. Place the potato skins in the fryer basket skin side down. Crack one egg into each potato skin.

6. Sprinkle ½ tablespoon of bacon pieces and ¼ cup of shredded cheese on top of each egg. Sprinkle with salt and pepper to taste.

7. Air fry until the yolk is slightly runny, 5 to 6 minutes, or until the yolk is fully cooked, 7 to 10 minutes.

Make it Even Lower Calorie: Use reduced-calorie cheddar cheese.

Per Serving

Calories: 338; Total Fat: 15g; Saturated Fat: 8g; Cholesterol: 214mg; Carbohydrates: 35g; Protein: 17g; Fiber: 3g; Sodium: 301mg

Greek Frittata

PREP TIME: 10 MINUTES / **COOK TIME:** 20 MINUTES / **SERVES** 4 (MAKES 2 FRITTATAS) / 350°F

A frittata is an egg-based Italian dish that is very easy to customize. Almost any kind of vegetable, meat, or cheese can be mixed with the eggs to create a unique one-dish meal. Here, I'm making it Greek-style with tomatoes and feta cheese, one of my favorite combinations.

GLUTEN-FREE

VEGETARIAN

Olive oil
5 eggs
¼ teaspoon salt
⅛ teaspoon freshly ground black pepper
1 cup baby spinach leaves, shredded
½ cup halved grape tomatoes
½ cup crumbled feta cheese

1. Spray a small round air fryer-friendly pan with olive oil.

2. In a medium bowl, whisk together eggs, salt, and pepper and whisk to combine.

3. Add the spinach and stir to combine.

4. Pour ½ cup of the egg mixture into the pan.

5. Sprinkle ¼ cup of the tomatoes and ¼ cup of the feta on top of the egg mixture.

6. Cover the pan with aluminum foil and secure it around the edges.

7. Place the pan carefully into the fryer basket.

8. Air fry for 12 minutes.

9. Remove the foil from the pan and cook until the eggs are set, 5 to 7 minutes.

10. Remove the frittata from the pan and place on a serving platter. Repeat with the remaining ingredients.

Air Fry Like a Pro: Spraying the pan beforehand makes it easy to remove the frittata so you can use the pan to make the second frittata. Alternatively, you could use two pans.

Per Serving (half of 1 frittata)

Calories: 146; Total Fat: 10g; Saturated Fat: 5g; Cholesterol: 249mg; Carbohydrates: 3g; Protein: 11g; Fiber: 1g; Sodium: 454mg

Mini Shrimp Frittata

PREP TIME: 15 MINUTES / **COOK TIME:** 20 MINUTES / **SERVES** 4 / 350°F

Baby shrimp make this recipe a breeze and they are the perfect size for an individual frittata. Shrimp pack a nice punch of flavor along with much-needed protein. Try serving this for Sunday brunch.

GLUTEN-FREE

1 teaspoon olive oil, plus more for spraying
½ small red bell pepper, finely diced
1 teaspoon minced garlic
1 (4-ounce) can of tiny shrimp, drained
Salt
Freshly ground black pepper
4 eggs, beaten
4 teaspoons ricotta cheese

1. Spray four ramekins with olive oil.

2. In a medium skillet over medium-low heat, heat 1 teaspoon of olive oil. Add the bell pepper and garlic and sauté until the pepper is soft, about 5 minutes

3. Add the shrimp, season with salt and pepper, and cook until warm, 1 to 2 minutes. Remove from the heat.

4. Add the eggs and stir to combine.

5. Pour one quarter of the mixture into each ramekin.

6. Place 2 ramekins in the fryer basket and cook for 6 minutes.

7. Remove the fryer basket from the air fryer and stir the mixture in each ramekin. Top each fritatta with 1 teaspoon of ricotta cheese. Return the fryer basket to the air fryer and cook until eggs are set and the top is lightly browned, 4 to 5 minutes.

8. Repeat with the remaining two ramekins.

Per Serving

Calories: 114; Total Fat: 7g; Saturated Fat: 2g; Cholesterol: 291mg; Carbohydrates: 1g; Protein: 12g; Fiber: <1g; Sodium: 291mg

Spinach and Mushroom Mini Quiche

PREP TIME: 10 MINUTES / **COOK TIME:** 15 MINUTES / **SERVES** 4 / 350°F

Spinach is considered a superfood, and the more we can incorporate it into recipes, the more nutrients we are feeding our bodies. Mushrooms are the best source of the antioxidant selenium you can find in the produce aisle. Adding both of these uber nutritious vegetables to the mini quiches results in a very healthy breakfast. This is an easy recipe to double or triple, so I suggest you do so and freeze the extras for a quick reheatable lunch.

GLUTEN-FREE

VEGETARIAN

1 teaspoon olive oil, plus more for spraying
1 cup coarsely chopped mushrooms
1 cup fresh baby spinach, shredded
4 eggs, beaten
½ cup shredded Cheddar cheese
½ cup shredded mozzarella cheese
¼ teaspoon salt
¼ teaspoon black pepper

1. Spray 4 silicone baking cups with olive oil and set aside.

2. In a medium sauté pan over medium heat, warm 1 teaspoon of olive oil. Add the mushrooms and sauté until soft, 3 to 4 minutes.

3. Add the spinach and cook until wilted, 1 to 2 minutes. Set aside.

4. In a medium bowl, whisk together the eggs, Cheddar cheese, mozzarella cheese, salt, and pepper.

5. Gently fold the mushrooms and spinach into the egg mixture.

6. Pour ¼ of the mixture into each silicone baking cup.

7. Place the baking cups into the fryer basket and air fry for 5 minutes. Stir the mixture in each ramekin slightly and air fry until the egg has set, an additional 3 to 5 minutes.

Make it Even Lower Calorie: Use all mozzarella cheese, which is lower in calories, instead of Cheddar cheese.

Per Serving

Calories: 183; Total Fat: 13g; Saturated Fat: 7g; Cholesterol: 206mg; Carbohydrates: 3g; Protein: 14g; Fiber: 1g; Sodium: 411mg

Italian Egg Cups

PREP TIME: 5 MINUTES / **COOK TIME:** 10 MINUTES / **SERVES** 4 / 350°F

A similar dish to shakshuka, a traditional Mediterranean specialty, these egg cups make a hearty brunch entrée. When buying marinara make sure to look for a sauce with no added sugar. The individual ramekins make it easy to control portion size.

GLUTEN-FREE

VEGETARIAN

Olive oil
1 cup marinara sauce
4 eggs
4 tablespoons shredded mozzarella cheese
4 teaspoons grated Parmesan cheese
Salt
Freshly ground black pepper
Chopped fresh basil, for garnish

1. Lightly spray 4 individual ramekins with olive oil.

2. Pour ¼ cup of marinara sauce into each ramekin.

3. Crack one egg into each ramekin on top of the marinara sauce.

4. Sprinkle 1 tablespoon of mozzarella and 1 tablespoon of Parmesan on top of each egg. Season with salt and pepper.

5. Cover each ramekin with aluminum foil. Place two of the ramekins in the fryer basket.

6. Air fry for 5 minutes and remove the aluminum foil. Air fry until the top is lightly browned and the egg white is cooked, another 2 to 4 minutes. If you prefer the yolk to be firmer, cook for 3 to 5 more minutes.

7. Repeat with the remaining two ramekins. Garnish with basil and serve.

Per Serving

Calories: 135; Total Fat: 8g; Saturated Fat: 3g; Cholesterol: 191mg; Carbohydrates: 6g; Protein: 10g; Fiber: 1g; Sodium: 407mg

Mexican Breakfast Pepper Rings

PREP TIME: 5 MINUTES / **COOK TIME:** 10 MINUTES / **SERVES** 4 / 350°F

Brightly colored bell peppers and a pop of salsa make a pretty contrast against the whiteness of the eggs. Starting the day with a protein-packed, low-calorie breakfast like this one is an ideal choice when you know you will be eating a more indulgent lunch or dinner later on.

DAIRY-FREE

GLUTEN-FREE

VEGETARIAN

Olive oil
1 large red, yellow, or orange bell pepper, cut into four ¾-inch rings
4 eggs
Salt
Freshly ground black pepper
2 teaspoons salsa

1. Lightly spray a small round air fryer–friendly pan with olive oil.

2. Place 2 bell pepper rings on the pan. Crack one egg into each bell pepper ring. Season with salt and black pepper.

3. Spoon ½ teaspoon of salsa on top of each egg.

4. Place the pan in the fryer basket. Air fry until the yolk is slightly runny, 5 to 6 minutes or until the yolk is fully cooked, 8 to 10 minutes.

5. Repeat with the remaining 2 pepper rings. Serve hot.

Pair It With: Turkey sausage or turkey bacon make this a heartier morning meal.

Air Fry Like a Pro: Use a silicone spatula to easily move the rings from the pan to your plate.

Per Serving

Calories: 84; Total Fat: 5g; Saturated Fat: 2g; Cholesterol: 186mg; Carbohydrates: 3g; Protein: 7g; Fiber: 1g; Sodium: 83mg

Cajun Breakfast Muffins

PREP TIME: 10 MINUTES / **COOK TIME:** 10 MINUTES / **SERVES** 6 / 350°F

I love grab-and-go breakfast options, and these Cajun-spiced muffins and can be reheated throughout the week for a quick morning meal. The combination of proteins and carbohydrates makes them filling and satisfying without raising the calories much. If you don't care for Cajun seasoning, use salt and pepper or an all-purpose seasoned salt.

GLUTEN-FREE

Olive oil
4 eggs, beaten
2¼ cups frozen hash browns, thawed
1 cup diced ham
½ cup shredded Cheddar cheese
½ teaspoon Cajun seasoning

1. Lightly spray 12 silicone muffin cups with olive oil.

2. In a medium bowl, mix together the eggs, hash browns, ham, Cheddar cheese, and Cajun seasoning in a medium bowl.

3. Spoon a heaping 1½ tablespoons of hash brown mixture into each muffin cup.

4. Place the muffin cups in the fryer basket.

5. Air fry until the muffins are golden brown on top and the center has set up, 8 to 10 minutes.

Make It Even Lower Calorie: Reduce or eliminate the cheese.

Per Serving (2 muffins)

Calories: 178; Total Fat: 9g; Saturated Fat: 4g; Cholesterol: 145mg; Carbohydrates: 13g; Protein: 11g; Fiber: 2g; Sodium: 467mg

Hearty Blueberry Oatmeal

PREP TIME: 10 MINUTES / **COOK TIME:** 25 MINUTES / **SERVES** 6 / 360°F

Blueberries are low in calories, high in nutrients, and one of the most powerful antioxidant foods. They are an excellent choice for people trying to add healthier foods to their diets. This oatmeal dish has a big blueberry flavor with just a hint of sweetness from the honey and cinnamon-sugar topping.

DAIRY-FREE

VEGETARIAN

1½ cups quick oats
1¼ teaspoons ground cinnamon, divided
½ teaspoon baking powder
Pinch salt
1 cup unsweetened vanilla almond milk
¼ cup honey
1 teaspoon vanilla extract
1 egg, beaten
2 cups blueberries
Olive oil
1½ teapoons sugar, divided
6 tablespoons low-fat whipped topping (optional)

1. In a large bowl, mix together the oats, 1 teaspoon of cinnamon, baking powder, and salt.

2. In a medium bowl, whisk together the almond milk, honey, vanilla and egg.

3. Pour the liquid ingredients into the oats mixture and stir to combine. Fold in the blueberries.

4. Lightly spray a round air fryer–friendly pan with oil.

5. Add half the blueberry mixture to the pan.

6. Sprinkle ⅛ teaspoon of cinnamon and ½ teaspoon sugar over the top.

7. Cover the pan with aluminum foil and place gently in the fryer basket.

8. Air fry for 20 minutes. Remove the foil and air fry for an additional 5 minutes. Transfer the mixture to a shallow bowl.

9. Repeat with the remaining blueberry mixture, ½ teaspoon of sugar, and ⅛ teaspoon of cinnamon.

10. To serve, spoon into bowls and top with whipped topping.

Per Serving

Calories: 170; Total Fat: 3g; Saturated Fat: 1g; Cholesterol: 97mg; Carbohydrates: 34g; Protein: 4g; Fiber: 4g; Sodium: 97mg

Banana Bread Pudding

PREP TIME: 10 MINUTES / **COOK TIME:** 20 MINUTES / **SERVES** 4 / 350°F

This healthier version of French toast is packed full of fiber for a hearty start to your day. The use of whole-grain bread versus white bread increases the nutritional value tremendously. Protein from the peanut butter will keep your hunger at bay until lunchtime.

VEGETARIAN

Olive oil
2 medium ripe bananas, mashed
½ cup low-fat milk
2 tablespoons peanut butter
2 tablespoons maple syrup
1 teaspoon ground cinnamon
1 teaspoon vanilla extract
2 slices whole-grain bread, torn into bite-sized pieces
¼ cup quick oats

1. Lightly spray four individual ramekins or one air fryer–safe baking dish with olive oil.

2. In a large mixing bowl, combine the bananas, milk, peanut butter, maple syrup, cinnamon, and vanilla. Using an electric mixer or whisk, mix until fully combined.

3. Add the bread pieces and stir to coat in the liquid mixture.

4. Add the oats and stir until everything is combined.

5. Transfer the mixture to the baking dish or divide between the ramekins. Cover with aluminum foil.

6. Place 2 ramekins in the fryer basket and air fry until heated through, 10 to 12 minutes.

7. Remove the foil and cook for 6 to 8 more minutes.

8. Repeat with the remaining 2 ramekins.

Make It Even Lower Calorie: Reduce the calories by using sugar-free maple syrup or by replacing the peanut butter with PB2 (powdered peanut butter). Combine 4 tablespoons of powdered peanut butter with 2 tablespoons of water to equal 2 tablespoons of peanut butter.

Per Serving

Calories: 212; Total Fat: 6g; Saturated Fat: 2g; Cholesterol: 2mg; Carbohydrates: 38g; Protein: 6g; Fiber: 5g; Sodium: 112mg

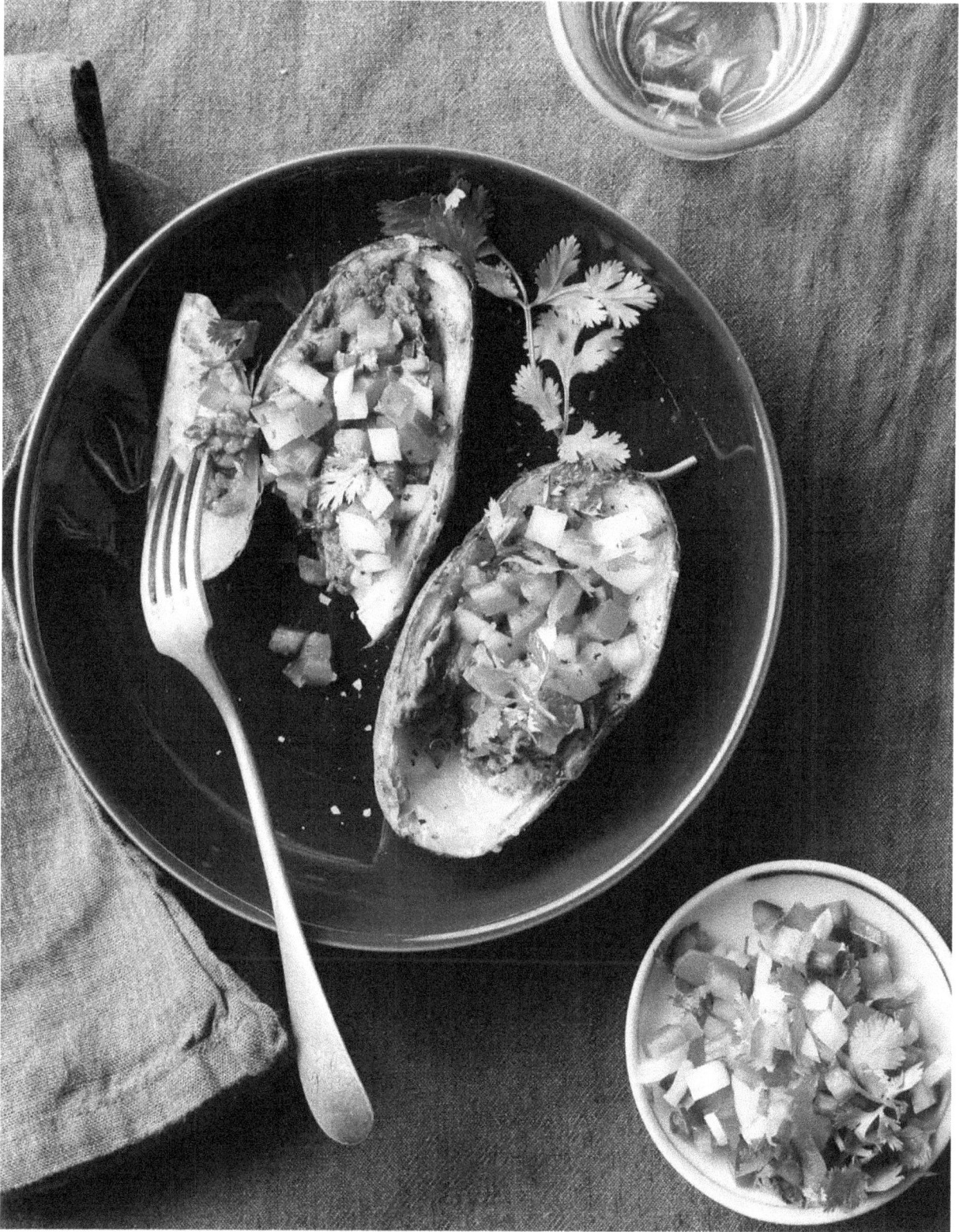

MEXICAN POTATO SKINS

CHAPTER 4

Healthy Snacks

Garlic Edamame

Spicy Chickpeas

Black Bean Corn Dip

Crunchy Tex-Mex Tortilla Chips

Egg Roll Pizza Sticks

Cajun Zucchini Chips

Mexican Potato Skins

Crispy Old Bay Chicken Wings

Cinnamon Apple Chips

Cinnamon and Sugar Peaches

Garlic Edamame

PREP TIME: 5 MINUTES / **COOK TIME:** 10 MINUTES / **SERVES** 4 / 375°F

Edamame are young green soybeans, and they make a tasty low-calorie snack. To eat them, simply squeeze the beans out of the pod directly into your mouth. Edamame are a wonderful source of protein and healthy fats, and you can season them a number of ways including the very simple method in this recipe.

DAIRY-FREE

GLUTEN-FREE

VEGETARIAN

Olive oil
1 (16-ounce) bag frozen edamame in pods
½ teaspoon salt
½ teaspoon garlic salt
¼ teaspoon freshly ground black pepper
½ teaspoon red pepper flakes (optional)

1. Spray a fryer basket lightly with olive oil.

2. In a medium bowl, add the frozen edamame and lightly spray with olive oil. Toss to coat.

3. In a small bowl, mix together the salt, garlic salt, black pepper, and red pepper flakes (if using). Add the mixture to the edamame and toss until evenly coated.

4. Place half the edamame in the fryer basket. Do not overfill the basket.

5. Air fry for 5 minutes. Shake the basket and cook until the edamame is starting to brown and get crispy, 3 to 5 more minutes.

6. Repeat with the remaining edamame and serve immediately.

Pair It With: These make a nice side dish to almost any meal.

Air Fry Like a Pro: If you use fresh edamame, reduce the air fry time by 2 to 3 minutes to avoid overcooking. Air-fried edamame do not retain their crisp texture, so it's best to eat them right after cooking.

Per Serving

Calories: 100; Total Fat: 3g; Saturated Fat: 0g; Cholesterol: 0mg; Carbohydrates: 9g; Protein: 8g; Fiber: 4g; Sodium: 496mg

Spicy Chickpeas

PREP TIME: 5 MINUTES / **COOK TIME:** 20 MINUTES / **SERVES** 4 / 390°F

Chickpeas, also known as garbanzo beans, have a mild flavor that pairs well with the spices in this recipe. I use a lot of canned chickpeas, which are precooked and can quickly be turned into really delicious snacks. They are high in fiber and protein and low on the glycemic index, making them a snack that's good for you.

DAIRY-FREE

GLUTEN-FREE

VEGETARIAN

Olive oil
½ teaspoon ground cumin
½ teaspoon chili powder
¼ teaspoon cayenne pepper
¼ teaspoon salt
1 (19-ounce) can chickpeas, drained and rinsed

1. Spray a fryer basket lightly with olive oil.

2. In a small bowl, combine the cumin, chili powder, cayenne pepper, and salt.

3. In a medium bowl, add the chickpeas and lightly spray them with olive oil. Add the spice mixture and toss until coated evenly.

4. Transfer the chickpeas to the fryer basket. Air fry until the chickpeas reach your desired level of crunchiness, 15 to 20 minutes, making sure to shake the basket every 5 minutes.

Air Fry Like a Pro: I find 20 minutes to be the sweet spot for very crunchy chickpeas. If you prefer them less crispy, cook for about 15 minutes. These make a great vehicle for experimenting with different seasoning mixes such as Chinese 5-spice, a mixture of curry and turmeric, or herbes de Provence.

Per Serving

Calories: 122; Total Fat: 1g; Saturated Fat: 0g; Cholesterol: 0mg; Carbohydrates: 22g; Protein: 6g; Fiber: 6g; Sodium: 152mg

Black Bean Corn Dip

PREP TIME: 10 MINUTES / **COOK TIME:** 10 MINUTES / **SERVES** 4 / 325°F

I love recipes that I can throw together quickly for last-minute guests or parties. This flavorful and hearty dip is a family favorite, and whoever you serve it to will love it too. It's easy to spice up using medium or hot salsa or adding a pinch of cayenne pepper. Keep the calories low by eating this with Cajun Zucchini Chips or serve with cut-up fresh veggies instead of traditional chips.

GLUTEN-FREE

VEGETARIAN

½ (15-ounce) can black beans, drained and rinsed
½ (15-ounce) can corn, drained and rinsed
¼ cup chunky salsa
2 ounces reduced-fat cream cheese, softened
¼ cup shredded reduced-fat Cheddar cheese
½ teaspoon ground cumin
½ teaspoon paprika
Salt
Freshly ground black pepper

1. In a medium bowl, mix together the black beans, corn, salsa, cream cheese, Cheddar cheese, cumin, and paprika. Season with salt and pepper and stir until well combined.

2. Spoon the mixture into an air fryer–safe baking dish.

3. Place baking dish in the fryer basket and air fry until heated through, about 10 minutes.

4. Serve hot.

Pair It With: If you're really craving chips, serve the dip with Crunchy Tex-Mex Tortilla Chips.

Air Fry Like a Pro: This isn't a traditional air fryer recipe, but I wanted to show you how versatile the air fryer can be. This dip is quick to put together and there is no need to heat up the whole kitchen by baking it in a traditional oven.

Per Serving

Calories: 129; Total Fat: 4g; Saturated Fat: 2g; Cholesterol: 11mg; Carbohydrates: 18g; Protein: 6g; Fiber: 4g; Sodium: 200mg

Crunchy Tex-Mex Tortilla Chips

PREP TIME: 5 MINUTES / **COOK TIME:** 5 MINUTES / **SERVES** 4 / 375°F

If you crave crunchy, seasoned chips but don't want all the unhealthy ingredients found in store-bought bags, give these a try. The blend of Tex-Mex–inspired spices like cumin, chili powder, and paprika bring a burst of flavor to each bite. Store any leftover chips in an airtight container to retain that crispy, fresh taste.

DAIRY-FREE

VEGETARIAN

Olive oil
½ teaspoon salt
½ teaspoon ground cumin
½ teaspoon chili powder
½ teaspoon paprika
Pinch cayenne pepper
8 (6-inch) corn tortillas, each cut into 6 wedges

1. Spray fryer basket lightly with olive oil.

2. In a small bowl, combine the salt, cumin, chili powder, paprika, and cayenne pepper.

3. Place the tortilla wedges in the fryer basket in a single layer. Spray the tortillas lightly with oil and sprinkle with some of the seasoning mixture. You will need to cook the tortillas in batches.

4. Air fry for 2 to 3 minutes. Shake the basket and cook until the chips are light brown and crispy, an additional 2 to 3 minutes. Watch the chips closely so they do not burn.

Pair It With: Serve with a simple salsa or the Black Bean Corn Dip for an even heartier snack.

Make It Gluten-Free: This recipe works just as well with gluten-free corn tortillas. Read the ingredients list on the package carefully to make sure they are gluten-free.

Air Fry Like a Pro: Use a pizza cutter to cut the tortillas quickly and easily. The chips will cook quickly, and the result is a very crunchy chip that gets crispier as it cools. Check on them every couple of minutes to make sure they're cooked to your taste.

Per Serving

Calories: 116; Total Fat: 2g; Saturated Fat: <1g; Cholesterol: 0mg; Carbohydrates: 24g; Protein: 3g; Fiber: 4g; Sodium: 321mg

Egg Roll Pizza Sticks

PREP TIME: 10 MINUTES / **COOK TIME:** 5 MINUTES / **SERVES** 4 / 375°F

A perfect balance of cheese, pepperoni, and crunch make these a crave-worthy snack, and using turkey pepperoni keeps the calories reasonable. I love serving them at parties because they look great on a platter with a bowl of warm marinara set in the center for dipping.

Olive oil
8 pieces reduced-fat string cheese
8 egg roll wrappers
24 slices turkey pepperoni
Marinara sauce, for dipping (optional)

1. Spray a fryer basket lightly with olive oil. Fill a small bowl with water.

2. Place each egg roll wrapper diagonally on a work surface. It should look like a diamond.

3. Place 3 slices of turkey pepperoni in a vertical line down the center of the wrapper.

4. Place 1 mozzarella cheese stick on top of the turkey pepperoni.

5. Fold the top and bottom corners of the egg roll wrapper over the cheese stick.

6. Fold the left corner over the cheese stick and roll the cheese stick up to resemble a spring roll. Dip a finger in the water and seal the edge of the roll

7. Repeat with the rest of the pizza sticks.

8. Place them in the fryer basket in a single layer, making sure to leave a little space between each one. Lightly spray the pizza sticks with oil. You may need to cook these in batches.

9. Air fry until the pizza sticks are lightly browned and crispy, about 5 minutes.

10. These are best served hot while the cheese is melted. Accompany with a small bowl of marinara sauce, if desired.

Air Fry Like a Pro: Overcooking will lead to the cheese melting and oozing out of the egg roll wrapper. If you'd like to ramp up the flavor, sprinkle the egg roll wrapper with a pinch of garlic powder before cooking.

Per Serving

Calories: 362; Total Fat: 8g; Saturated Fat: 4g; Cholesterol: 43mg; Carbohydrates: 40g; Protein: 23g; Fiber: 1g; Sodium: 1,026mg

Cajun Zucchini Chips

PREP TIME: 10 MINUTES / **COOK TIME:** 15 MINUTES / **SERVES** 4 / 370°F

Zucchini is packed with nutrients like vitamin A, vitamin C, potassium, fiber, and folate. Air frying zucchini slices turns them into crispy chips, and they are a wonderful substitute for processed snack foods. Remember, zucchini is full of water and they will shrink when cooked, so you may want to double or triple this recipe because they are so good, they won't last! If you have a mandolin, it will be easy to cut the zucchini very thin, though a sharp knife will work as well.

DAIRY-FREE

GLUTEN-FREE

VEGETARIAN

Olive oil
2 large zucchini, cut into ⅛-inch-thick slices
2 teaspoons Cajun seasoning

1. Spray a fryer basket lightly with olive oil.

2. Put the zucchini slices in a medium bowl and spray them generously with olive oil.

3. Sprinkle the Cajun seasoning over the zucchini and stir to make sure they are evenly coated with oil and seasoning.

4. Place slices in a single layer in the fryer basket, making sure not to overcrowd. You will need to cook these in several batches.

5. Air fry for 8 minutes. Flip the slices over and air fry until they are as crisp and brown as you prefer, an additional 7 to 8 minutes.

Air Fry Like a Pro: In order to achieve the best result, it is important not to overcrowd the fryer basket. The zucchini chips turn out best if there is room for the air to circulate around each slice. You can add cooking time if you like very brown and crunchy zucchini chips.

Per Serving

Calories: 26; Total Fat: <1g; Saturated Fat: <1g; Cholesterol: 0mg; Carbohydrates: 5g; Protein: 2g; Fiber: 2g; Sodium: 286mg

Mexican Potato Skins

PREP TIME: 10 MINUTES / **COOK TIME:** 55 MINUTES / **SERVES** 6 / 400°F

Potato skins are a party favorite, and this recipe brings protein and extra flavor to the festivities along with an extra crispy touch to the skins from air frying. Although the calories are lower than usual because most of the insides have been removed and replaced with black beans and salsa, potatoes are best eaten in moderation; so make this only occasionally for a special celebration.

GLUTEN-FREE

VEGETARIAN

Olive oil
6 medium russet potatoes, scrubbed
Salt
Freshly ground black pepper
1 cup fat-free refried black beans
1 tablespoon taco seasoning
½ cup salsa
¾ cup reduced-fat shredded Cheddar cheese

1. Spray a fryer basket lightly with olive oil.

2. Spray the potatoes lightly with oil and season with salt and pepper. Pierce each potato a few times with a fork.

3. Place the potatoes in the fryer basket. Air fry until fork tender, 30 to 40 minutes. The cooking time will depend on the size of the potatoes. You can cook the potatoes in the microwave or a standard oven, but they won't get the same lovely crispy skin they will get in the air fryer.

4. While the potatoes are cooking, in a small bowl, mix together the beans and taco seasoning. Set aside until the potatoes are cool enough to handle.

5. Cut each potato in half lengthwise. Scoop out most of the insides, leaving about ¼ inch in the skins so the potato skins hold their shape.

6. Season the insides of the potato skins with salt and black pepper. Lightly

spray the insides of the potato skins with oil. You may need to cook them in batches.

7. Place them into the fryer basket, skin side down, and air fry until crisp and golden, 8 to 10 minutes.

8. Transfer the skins to a work surface and spoon ½ tablespoon of seasoned refried black beans into each one. Top each with 2 teaspoons salsa and 1 tablespoon shredded Cheddar cheese.

9. Place filled potato skins in the fryer basket in a single layer. Lightly spray with oil.

10. Air fry until the cheese is melted and bubbly, 2 to 3 minutes.

Make It Even Lower Calorie: Omit the shredded cheese.

Per Serving

Calories: 245; Total Fat: 3g; Saturated Fat: 2g; Cholesterol: 10mg; Carbohydrates: 46g; Protein: 10g; Fiber: 5g; Sodium: 461mg

Crispy Old Bay Chicken Wings

PREP TIME: 10 MINUTES / **COOK TIME:** 15 MINUTES / **SERVES** 4 / 400°F

Chicken wings are an American favorite, but deep-fried wings are loaded with unhealthy fats and calories. And many people drive the calories even higher by drenching their wings in high-calorie sauces. This recipe doesn't need the additional sauce because they will completely satisfy you without it. Cooking the wings in the air fryer will become a regular occurrence for you because it is so easy to do, and the results are incredibly crispy and delicious.

DAIRY-FREE

GLUTEN-FREE

Olive oil
2 tablespoons Old Bay seasoning
2 teaspoons baking powder
2 teaspoons salt
2 pounds chicken wings

1. Spray a fryer basket lightly with olive oil.

2. In a large zip-top plastic bag, mix together the Old Bay seasoning, baking powder, and salt.

3. Pat the wings dry with paper towels.

4. Place the wings in the zip-top bag, seal, and toss with the seasoning mixture until evenly coated.

5. Place the seasoned wings in the fryer basket in a single layer. Lightly spray with olive oil. You may need to cook them in batches.

6. Air fry for 7 minutes. Turn the wings over, lightly spray them with olive oil, and air fry until the wings are crispy and lightly browned, 5 to 8 more minutes. Using a meat thermometer, check to make sure the internal temperature is 165°F or higher.

Per Serving

Calories: 501; Total Fat: 36g; Saturated Fat: 10g; Cholesterol: 170mg; Carbohydrates: 1g; Protein: 42g; Fiber: 0g; Sodium: 2,527mg

Cinnamon Apple Chips

PREP TIME: 10 MINUTES / **COOK TIME:** 10 MINUTES / **SERVES** 4 / 350°F

The delicious smell of apples and cinnamon will waft through the house as you cook these sweet, crunchy treats. This is a great way to use apples that are on the verge of being too ripe to eat. There's no sugar added, and by leaving the peels on, you'll get a nutritional boost of soluble fiber and vitamins.

DAIRY-FREE

GLUTEN-FREE

VEGETARIAN

Olive oil
2 apples, any variety, cored, cut in half, and cut into thin slices
2 heaped teaspoons ground cinnamon

1. Spray a fryer basket lightly with oil.

2. In a medium bowl, toss the apple slices with the cinnamon until evenly coated.

3. Place the apple slices in the fryer basket in a single layer. You may need to cook them in batches.

4. Air fry for 4 to 5 minutes. Shake the basket and cook until crispy, another 4 to 5 minutes.

Air Fry Like a Pro: Cook time will depend on the thickness of the apple slices and how crispy you want the slices to be. It is fine to remove slices from the basket that are done to your liking to avoid scorching. Add additional cook time for slices that don't have a "dehydrated" look yet. If slices stick together just separate them and continue cooking. The apple slices will get crispier as they cool.

Per Serving

Calories: 39; Total Fat: <1g; Saturated Fat: 0g; Cholesterol: 0mg; Carbohydrates: 11g; Protein: <1g; Fiber: 2g; Sodium: <1mg

Cinnamon and Sugar Peaches

PREP TIME: 10 MINUTES / **COOK TIME:** 13 MINUTES / **SERVES** 4 / 350°F

I remember picking peaches at an orchard with my family when I as a child. The velvety soft fruit has always been synonymous with dessert to me. Many peach desserts are loaded with calories and fat, but I've removed most of the sugar, relying on their inherent sweetness and a touch of cinnamon. They will curb your sweet tooth and keep you headed toward your goal.

DAIRY-FREE

GLUTEN-FREE

VEGETARIAN

Olive oil
2 tablespoons sugar
¼ teaspoon ground cinnamon
4 peaches, cut into wedges

1. Spray a fryer basket lightly with olive oil.

2. In a medium bowl, combine the sugar and cinnamon. Add the peaches and toss to coat evenly.

3. Place the peaches in a single layer in the fryer basket on their sides. You may need to cook them in batches.

4. Air fry for 5 minutes. Turn the peaches skin side down, lightly spray them with oil, and air fry until the peaches are lightly brown and caramelized, 5 to 8 more minutes.

Make it Even Lower Calorie: Use a zero calorie sugar substitute such as Nutrisweet or monk fruit sweetener instead of granulated sugar.

Air Fry Like a Pro: These do not get truly crispy, but rather they remain soft, sweet, and caramelized. They are truly delightful and make a wonderful dessert option.

Per Serving

Calories: 67; Total Fat: <1g; Saturated Fat: 0g; Cholesterol: 0mg; Carbohydrates: 17g; Protein: 1g; Fiber: 2g; Sodium: 0mg

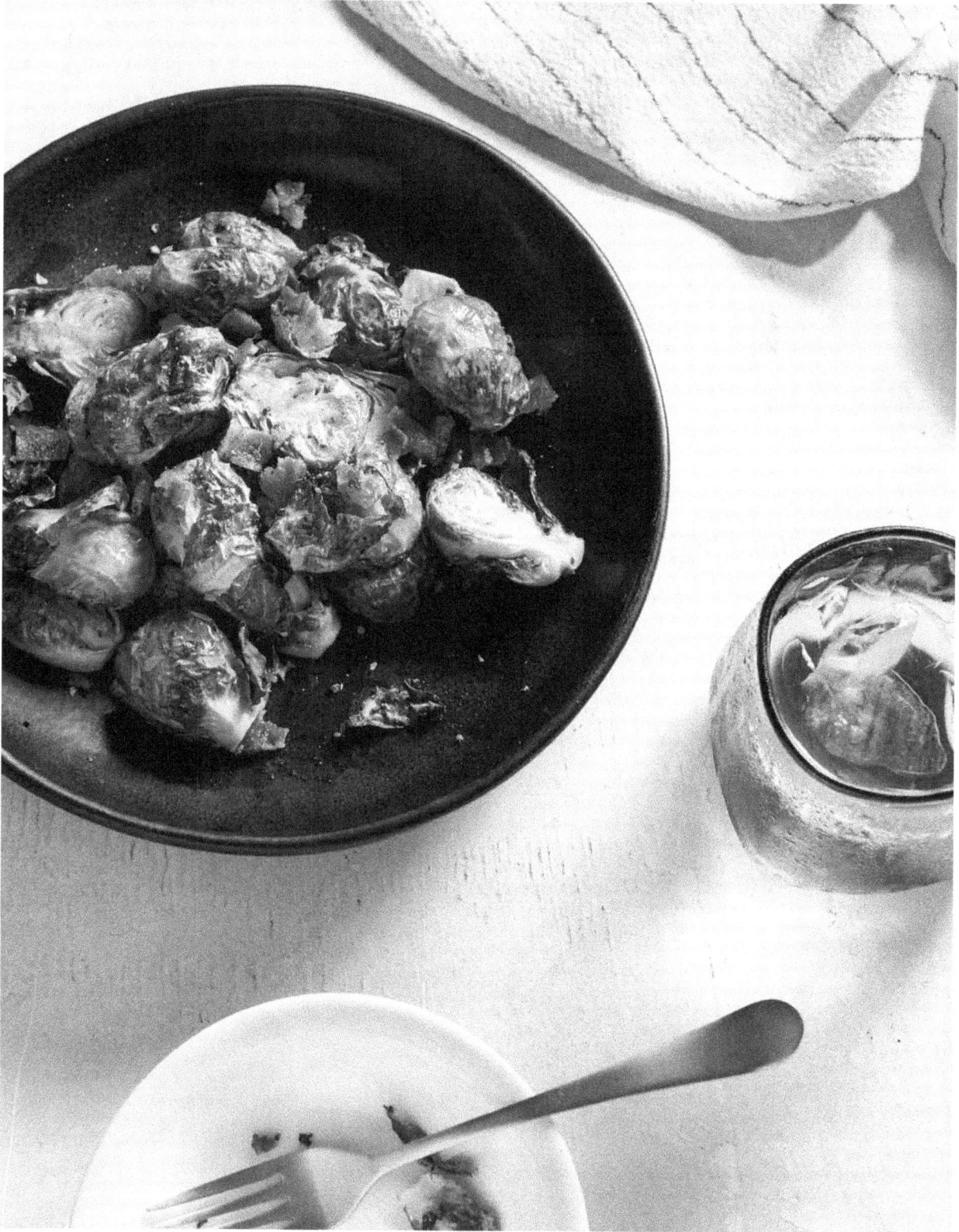

BACON ROASTED BRUSSELS SPROUTS

CHAPTER 5

Vegetables and Side Dishes

Avocado Fries

Spicy Dill Pickle Fries

Carrot Chips

Spicy Corn on the Cob

Bacon Roasted Brussels Sprouts

Cheesy Roasted Tomatoes

Crispy Breaded Bell Pepper Strips

Roasted "Everything Bagel" Broccolini

Sweet and Spicy Broccoli

Broccoli Cheese Tots

Spiced Balsamic Asparagus

Simple Roasted Cauliflower

Spinach and Cheese–Stuffed Mushrooms

Parmesan Green Beans

Green Beans and New Potatoes

Crunchy Hasselback Potatoes

Spicy Sweet Potatoes

Portobello Pizzas

Creole Seasoned Okra

Easy Homemade Veggie Burger

Avocado Fries

PREP TIME: 20 MINUTES / **COOK TIME:** 8 MINUTES / **SERVES** 6 / 350°F

Avocados are a superfood, high in fiber, and filled with a variety of vitamins and minerals. They are also a good source of healthy fat, and they are low in sugar. Like potatoes, avocados are higher in calories than other vegetables so they should be eaten in moderation.

`DAIRY-FREE`

`VEGETARIAN`

Olive oil
4 slightly under-ripe avocados, cut in half, pits removed
1½ cups whole-wheat panko bread crumbs
¾ teaspoon freshly ground black pepper
1½ teaspoons paprika
¾ teaspoon salt
3 eggs

1. Spray a fryer basket lightly with olive oil.

2. Carefully remove the skin from the avocado leaving the flesh intact. Cut each avocado half lengthwise into 5 to 6 slices. Set aside.

3. In a small bowl, mix together the panko bread crumbs, black pepper, paprika, and salt.

4. In a separate small bowl, whisk the eggs.

5. Coat each avocado slice in the egg and then in the panko mixture, pressing the panko mixture gently into the avocado so it sticks.

6. Place the avocado slices in the fryer basket in a single layer. Lightly spray with olive oil. You may need to cook them in batches.

7. Air fry for 3 to 4 minutes. Turn the slices over and spray lightly with olive oil.

8. Air fry until light brown and crispy, 3 to 4 more minutes.

Air Fry Like a Pro: Make sure to leave a little bit of space between the avocado slices so they get crispy all the way around.

Per Serving

Calories: 300; Total Fat: 20g; Saturated Fat: 3g; Cholesterol: 93mg; Carbohydrates: 25g; Protein: 9g; Fiber: 10g; Sodium: 358mg

Spicy Dill Pickle Fries

PREP TIME: 15 MINUTES / **COOK TIME:** 15 MINUTES / **SERVES** 4 / 400°F

If you love the taste of fried pickles, this recipe will become an instant favorite. The crispy crunch on the outside and the juicy pickle inside is the perfect contrast. The air fryer makes them lower calorie because you don't need so much oil to cook them. If you don't care for spicy pickles, just use regular dill spears instead.

DAIRY-FREE

VEGETARIAN

Olive oil
1 cup whole-wheat flour
1 teaspoon paprika
1 egg
1⅓ cups whole-wheat panko bread crumbs
1 (24-ounce) jar spicy dill pickle spears

1. Spray a fryer basket lightly with olive oil.

2. In a small, shallow bowl, combine the whole-wheat flour and paprika.

3. In another small, shallow bowl, whisk the egg.

4. Put the panko bread crumbs in another small.

5. Pat the pickle spears dry with paper towels.

6. Dip each pickle spear in the flour mixture, coat in the egg, and dredge in the panko bread crumbs.

7. Place each pickle spear in the fryer basket in a single layer, leaving a little space between each one. Spray the pickles lightly with olive oil. You may need to cook them in batches.

8. Air fry for 7 minutes. Turn the pickles over and cook until lightly browned and crispy, another 5 to 8 minutes.

Make It Even Lower Calorie: These spicy dill pickle fries are great dipped in ranch dressing. Instead of using traditional dressings that are high in calories and fat, buy a Greek yogurt-based ranch dip. This can save around 100 calories in just 2 tablespoons!

Per Serving

Calories: 233; Total Fat: 2g; Saturated Fat: 1g; Cholesterol: 47mg; Carbohydrates: 45g; Protein: 10g; Fiber: 7g; Sodium: 1,249mg

Carrot Chips

PREP TIME: 15 MINUTES / **COOK TIME:** 10 MINUTES / **SERVES** 4 / 390°F

It always amazes me how a simple root vegetable like a carrot can be transformed into a delicious snack using a little olive oil and seasoned salt plus some time in the air fryer. Carrots are a great source of beta carotene, fiber, potassium, and other antioxidants, and like many vegetables are very low in calories. Try making these as an after-school snack for your children; you may be surprised how much they enjoy eating them.

DAIRY-FREE

GLUTEN-FREE

VEGETARIAN

1 tablespoon olive oil plus more for spraying
4 to 5 medium carrots, trimmed
1 teaspoon seasoned salt

1. Spray a fryer basket lightly with olive oil.

2. Using a mandolin slicer set to the smallest setting or a sharp knife, cut the carrots into very thin slices.

3. In a medium bowl, toss the carrot slices with 1 tablespoon of olive oil and the seasoned salt.

4. Put half the carrots the fryer basket. Do not overcrowd the basket.

5. Air fry for 5 minutes. Shake the basket and cook until crispy, 3 to 5 additional minutes. The longer you cook the carrot slices, the crispier they will become. Watch closely because smaller slices could burn.

6. Repeat with the remaining carrots.

Air Fry Like a Pro: You can save time by purchasing a bag of crinkle cut carrots in the fresh produce section of the grocery store.

Per Serving

Calories: 55; Total Fat: 4g; Saturated Fat: 1g; Cholesterol: 0mg; Carbohydrates: 6g; Protein: 1g; Fiber: 2g; Sodium: 422mg

Spicy Corn on the Cob

PREP TIME: 10 MINUTES / **COOK TIME:** 16 MINUTES / **SERVES** 4 / 400°F

Corn on the cob on its own is around 100 calories. The problem has always been that people slather butter all over the it, doubling or tripling the calorie count. But when you make it in the air fryer you'll find that butter is not needed at all. Five sprays of olive oil are only around 10 calories and bring a wonderful flavor to this summertime favorite.

GLUTEN-FREE

VEGETARIAN

Olive oil
2 tablespoons grated Parmesan cheese
1 teaspoon chili powder
1 teaspoon garlic powder
1 teaspoon ground cumin
1 teaspoon paprika
1 teaspoon salt
¼ teaspoon cayenne pepper, optional
4 ears fresh corn, shucked

1. Spray a fryer basket lightly with olive oil.

2. In a small bowl, mix together the Parmesan cheese, chili powder, garlic powder, cumin, paprika, salt, and cayenne pepper.

3. Lightly spray the ears of corn with olive oil. Sprinkle them with the seasoning mixture.

4. Place the ears of corn in the fryer basket in a single layer. You may need to cook them in more than one batch.

5. Air fry for 7 minutes. Turn the corn over and air fry until lightly browned, 7 to 9 more minutes.

Make It Even Lower Calorie: This recipe is just as tasty without Parmesan, especially when the corn is super fresh and sweet.

Per Serving

Calories: 116; Total Fat: 2g; Saturated Fat: 1g; Cholesterol: 2mg; Carbohydrates: 23g; Protein: 5g; Fiber: 4g; Sodium: 652mg

Bacon Roasted Brussels Sprouts

PREP TIME: 10 MINUTES / **COOK TIME:** 10 MINUTES / **SERVES** 4 / 350°F

Brussel sprouts have never tasted so good than when they are cooked in the air fryer! They're also extremely healthy—1 cup contains less than 40 calories—and they're a great source of vitamins C and K.

DAIRY-FREE

GLUTEN-FREE

Olive oil
16 ounces fresh Brussels sprouts, trimmed and halved
1 tablespoon crumbled cooked bacon
2 teaspoons balsamic vinegar
1 teaspoon olive oil
1 teaspoon salt
1 teaspoon pepper

1. Spray a fryer basket lightly with olive oil.

2. In a medium bowl, toss the Brussels sprouts with the crumbled bacon, balsamic vinegar, olive oil, salt, and pepper.

3. Place the sprouts in the fryer basket. Air fry for 5 minutes. Shake the basket and lightly spray with the olive oil. Cook until the sprouts are fork-tender and lightly browned, another 3 to 5 minutes.

Air Fry Like a Pro: Brussels sprouts come in a variety of sizes. Cut large sprouts into quarters if necessary, and small ones don't need to be cut at all. The goal is to make them all the same size so they will cook evenly. When trimming, some of the leaves always come off, but that's OK—throw them in the fryer as well. They come out crisp and delicious with a flavor and texture similar to kale chips.

Make It Vegetarian: Omit the bacon.

Per Serving

Calories: 72; Total Fat: 2g; Saturated Fat: 1g; Cholesterol: 3mg; Carbohydrates: 11g; Protein: 5g; Fiber: 5g; Sodium: 651mg

Cheesy Roasted Tomatoes

PREP TIME: 10 MINUTES / **COOK TIME:** 6 MINUTES / **SERVES** 4 / 375°F

This recipe looks as good as it tastes with bright red tomatoes and crispy cheese. Make them for an appealing party snack or as an accompaniment to an entrée. Firm and meaty Roma tomatoes work best for this recipe because they hold up to air frying.

GLUTEN-FREE

VEGETARIAN

Olive oil
4 Roma tomatoes, cut into ½ inch slices
Salt
½ cup shredded mozzarella cheese
¼ cup shredded Parmesan cheese
Freshly ground black pepper
Parsley flakes

1. Spray a fryer basket lightly with olive oil.

2. Season the tomato slices lightly with salt.

3. Place the tomato slices in the fryer basket in a single layer. You may need to cook these in batches.

4. Sprinkle each tomato slice with 1 teaspoon of mozzarella cheese. Sprinkle ½ teaspoon of shredded Parmesan cheese on top of the mozzarella cheese on each tomato slice.

5. Season with black pepper and sprinkle parsley flakes over the top of the cheeses.

6. Air fry until the cheese is melted, bubbly, and lightly browned, 5 to 6 minutes.

Make It Even Lower Calorie: Omit the Parmesan cheese to reduce the calories a little.

Per Serving

Calories: 100; Total Fat: 5g; Saturated Fat: 3g; Cholesterol: 13mg; Carbohydrates: 8g; Protein: 7g; Fiber: 1g; Sodium: 195mg

Crispy Breaded Bell Pepper Strips

PREP TIME: 15 MINUTES / **COOK TIME:** 7 MINUTES / **SERVES** 4 / 400°F

Fried peppers are usually loaded in fat and calories. The breading is made with white flour, which is low in nutrients and fiber, and traditional frying uses large amounts of unhealthy vegetable oil. This air-fried rendition is just as tasty and much healthier and lower in calories. Try these as an alternative to French fries or chips when you are having burger night.

DAIRY-FREE

VEGETARIAN

Olive oil
⅔ cup whole-wheat panko bread crumbs
½ teaspoon paprika
½ teaspoon garlic powder
½ teaspoon salt
1 egg, beaten
2 red, orange, or yellow bell peppers, cut into ½-inch-thick slices

1. Spray a fryer basket lightly with olive oil.

2. In a medium shallow bowl, mix together the panko bread crumbs, paprika, garlic powder, and salt.

3. In a separate small shallow bowl, whisk the egg with 1½ teaspoons of water to make an egg wash.

4. Dip the bell pepper slices in the egg wash to coat, then dredge them in the panko bread crumbs until evenly coated.

5. Place the bell pepper slices in the fryer basket in a single layer. Lightly spray the bell pepper strips with oil. You may need to cook these in batches.

6. Air fry until lightly browned, 4 to 7 minutes.

7. Carefully remove from fryer basket to ensure the that the coating does not come off. Serve immediately.

Air Fry Like a Pro: If the bell pepper slices are not a uniform size they may not cook evenly. Very thin slices will burn easily and the panko bread crumbs will brown quickly in the air fryer.

Pair It With: These strips are great dipped in a low-calorie ranch dressing or a dip made from Greek yogurt.

Per Serving

Calories: 82; Total Fat: 1g; Saturated Fat: <1g; Cholesterol: 47mg; Carbohydrates: 14g; Protein: 4g; Fiber: 3g; Sodium: 325mg

Roasted "Everything Bagel" Broccolini

PREP TIME: 5 MINUTES / **COOK TIME:** 12 MINUTES / **SERVES** 4 / 375°F

Shake up your everyday vegetable routine with this easy, healthy dish made with broccolini. With long thin stalks and smaller florets than broccoli, broccolini is an excellent source of vitamin C and has only 35 calories per serving. It's irresistible when crisped up in the air fryer and combined with the complex flavors of everything bagel seasoning.

DAIRY-FREE

GLUTEN-FREE

VEGETARIAN

1½ teaspoons olive oil, plus more for spraying
1 pound broccolini
1 tablespoon everything bagel seasoning

1. Spray the fryer basket lightly with olive oil.

2. In a large bowl, toss the broccolini with the ½ tablespoon olive oil and everything bagel seasoning.

3. Place the broccolini in the fryer basket in a single layer. You may need to cook them in batches.

4. Air fry until the broccolini are tender and lightly browned, 8 to 12 minutes, making sure to shake the basket after 5 minutes of cooking. Repeat with any remaining broccolini.

Air Fry Like a Pro: It's important to coat the broccolini in olive oil so the ends don't char during the cooking process.

Pair It With: This flavorful dish makes a perfect side to Breaded Pork Cutlets or Beef and Mushroom Meatballs.

Per Serving

Calories: 62; Total Fat: 2g; Saturated Fat: <1g; Cholesterol: 0mg; Carbohydrates: 6g; Protein: 3g; Fiber: 3g; Sodium: 226mg

Sweet and Spicy Broccoli

PREP TIME: 10 MINUTES / **COOK TIME:** 20 MINUTES / **SERVES** 4 / 400°F

I love a side dish that can easily be paired with a lean protein and a high-quality carbohydrate to make a full meal in minutes. The combination of soy sauce and honey gives you the flavors found in classic stir-fries. Add a kick of heat with hot sauce, though you can leave that out for those who don't tolerate too much spiciness. If you want to reduce the sodium content in this recipe, use low-sodium soy sauce and a sodium-free salt substitute.

DAIRY-FREE

VEGETARIAN

½ teaspoon olive oil, plus more for spraying
1 pound fresh broccoli, cut into florets
½ tablespoon minced garlic
Salt
1½ tablespoons soy sauce
1 teaspoon white vinegar
2 teaspoons hot sauce or sriracha
1½ teaspoons honey
Freshly ground black pepper

1. Spray a fryer basket lightly with olive oil.

2. In a large bowl, toss the broccoli florets with ½ teaspoon of olive oil and the minced garlic. Season with salt.

3. Place the broccoli in the fryer basket in a single layer. Do not overcrowd the broccoli. You will need to cook this in more than one batch.

4. Air fry until lightly browned and crispy, 15 to 20 minutes, making sure to shake the basket every 5 minutes. Repeat for remaining broccoli.

5. While the broccoli is frying, in a small bowl, whisk together the soy sauce, white vinegar, hot sauce, honey, and black pepper. If the honey doesn't incorporate well, microwave the mixture for 10 to 20 seconds until the honey melts.

6. In a large bowl, toss the cooked broccoli with the sauce mixture. Season with additional salt and pepper, if desired. Serve immediately.

Pair It With: This is a bold, flavorful side dish that can be served over quinoa or brown rice and topped with the Chili-Lime Shrimp to make a satisfying one bowl meal. I like it with Seafood Spring Rolls or Teriyaki Chicken Bowls.

Air Fry Like a Pro: Some people like to cook their broccoli until it is almost charred while others prefer it to be just slightly browned on the edges. Watch the broccoli closely after the 10-minute mark so that it is cooked exactly how you want it.

Per Serving

Calories: 54; Total Fat: 1g; Saturated Fat: <1g; Cholesterol: 0mg; Carbohydrates: 10g; Protein: 4g; Fiber: 4g; Sodium: 419mg

Broccoli Cheese Tots

PREP TIME: 20 MINUTES / **COOK TIME:** 15 MINUTES / **SERVES** 4 / 375°F

Tater tots have always been a favorite of mine, but they shouldn't play a part in your weight-loss journey. In this recipe, though, I've replaced the carb-heavy potatoes with broccoli and whole wheat-bread crumbs, and mixed it with low-fat cheese to help hold it all together. Dip these in a low-sugar ketchup for a comforting side dish that won't knock you off the low-calorie wagon.

VEGETARIAN

Olive oil
12 ounces frozen broccoli, thawed and drained
1 large egg
1½ teaspoons minced garlic
¼ cup grated Parmesan cheese
¼ cup shredded reduced-fat sharp Cheddar cheese
½ cup seasoned whole-wheat bread crumbs
Salt
Freshly ground black pepper

1. Spray the fryer basket lightly with olive oil.

2. Gently squeeze the thawed broccoli to remove any excess liquid.

3. In a food processor, combine the broccoli, egg, garlic, Parmesan cheese, Cheddar cheese, bread crumbs, salt, and pepper and pulse until it resembles a coarse meal.

4. Using a tablespoon, scoop up the broccoli mixture and shape into 24 oval "tater tot" shapes.

5. Place the tots in the fryer basket in a single layer, being careful to space them a little bit apart. Lightly spray the tots with oil. You may need to cook them in batches.

6. Air fry for 6 to 7 minutes. Turn the tots over and cook for an additional 6 to 8 minutes or until lightly browned and crispy.

Make it Gluten-Free: Gluten-free bread crumbs will provide just as much crunch for these tots.

Air Fry Like a Pro: If you don't feel that your tots are getting crispy enough, spray with a little bit more olive oil halfway through the cooking time.

Per Serving (6 broccoli tots)

Calories: 128; Total Fat: 5g; Saturated Fat: 3g; Cholesterol: 56mg; Carbohydrates: 13g; Protein: 10g; Fiber: 4g; Sodium: 205mg

Spiced Balsamic Asparagus

PREP TIME: 15 MINUTES / **COOK TIME:** 10 MINUTES / **SERVES** 4 / 350°F

Asparagus is chock-full of healthy potential. One cup provides almost half of an adult's daily requirement for vitamin K. It's also high in folate, fiber, potassium, and antioxidants, and can even help support bone health. And with its strong flavor, it just needs some simple seasoning to make a delicious air-fried side dish. Just remember to trim the ends off, as they can be tough and woody.

DAIRY-FREE

GLUTEN-FREE

VEGETARIAN

4 tablespoons olive oil, plus more for spraying
4 tablespoons balsamic vinegar
1½ pounds asparagus, trimmed
Salt
Freshly ground black pepper

1. Spray a fryer basket lightly with olive oil.

2. In a medium shallow bowl, whisk together the 4 tablespoons of olive oil and balsamic vinegar to make a marinade.

3. Lay the asparagus in the bowl so they are completely covered by the oil and vinegar mixture and let marinate for 5 minutes.

4. Place the asparagus in a single layer in the air fryer and sprinkle with salt and pepper. You may need to cook them in batches.

5. Air fry for 5 minutes. Shake the basket and cook until the asparagus is tender and lightly browned, 3 to 5 more minutes.

Make It Even Lower Calorie: Although this recipe does include a larger amount of olive oil than other recipes in this book, most of it will remain in the bowl. It is important to completely coat the asparagus in the oil and vinegar mixture to prevent the asparagus from charring while cooking.

Per Serving

Calories: 167; Total Fat: 14g; Saturated Fat: 2g; Cholesterol: 0mg; Carbohydrates: 10g; Protein: 4g; Fiber: 4g; Sodium: 8mg

Simple Roasted Cauliflower

PREP TIME: 10 MINUTES / COOK TIME: 20 MINUTES / SERVES 4 / 400°F

Cauliflower is one of the most versatile vegetables due to its mild flavor. It tastes great with a wide range of different seasonings, and when air fried, delivers a satisfying, almost nutty flavor. It's also very low in calories but high in fiber and B vitamins.

DAIRY-FREE

GLUTEN-FREE

VEGETARIAN

Olive oil
1 large head cauliflower, broken into small florets
2 teaspoons smoked paprika
1 teaspoon garlic powder
Salt
Freshly ground black pepper

1. Spray a fryer basket lightly with olive oil.

2. In a large bowl, toss the cauliflower florets with the smoked paprika and garlic powder until well coated. Season with salt and pepper.

3. Put the cauliflower in the fryer basket. Lightly spray the florets with oil. You may need to cook them in batches.

4. Air fry until nicely browned and lightly crispy, 20 minutes, shaking the basket every 5 minutes. Serve hot.

Pair It With: This Simple Roasted Cauliflower goes well with almost any protein. Try creating a full meal by layering brown rice, roasted cauliflower, and Zesty Garlic Scallops. Top with a healthy dressing or sauce of your choice.

Air Fry Like a Pro: Always watch vegetables closely during the cooking process. Smaller florets will cook quicker than larger florets and may burn. It is fine to take the finished florets out of the basket and continue to cook the ones that aren't quite done yet.

Per Serving

Calories: 58; Total Fat: 1g; Saturated Fat: <1g; Cholesterol: 0mg; Carbohydrates: 12g; Protein: 4g; Fiber: 6g; Sodium: 64mg

Spinach and Cheese–Stuffed Mushrooms

PREP TIME: 15 MINUTES / **COOK TIME:** 10 MINUTES / **SERVES** 4 / 370°F

High in protein, mushrooms keep you full, while also providing a bounty of vitamins, minerals, and antioxidants. When buying them, look for mushrooms that are firm, dry, and unbruised. Store them in the refrigerator and don't clean them until just before you are ready cook.

VEGETARIAN

Olive oil
4 ounces reduced-fat cream cheese, softened
¾ cup shredded Italian blend cheese
¼ cup whole-wheat bread crumbs
1 egg
¼ teaspoon salt
¼ teaspoon freshly ground black pepper
1 cup fresh baby spinach, chopped
20 large mushrooms, stems removed

1. Spray a fryer basket lightly with olive oil.

2. In a medium bowl, use an electric mixer to combine the cream cheese, Italian blend cheese, bread crumbs, egg, salt, and pepper.

3. Add the spinach and stir with a spoon to combine.

4. Spoon the mixture into each mushroom, pressing the mixture into the mushroom and leaving a little bit popping out of the top.

5. Place the stuffed mushrooms in a single layer in the fryer basket. Spray lightly with olive oil. You may need to cook these in more than one batch.

6. Air fry until the mushrooms have started to brown lightly and the cheese is lightly brown on top, 7 to 10 minutes.

Pair It With: Stuffed mushrooms are a wonderful appetizer for parties, but they also work as a great side dish. Pair these with Beef Roll-Ups for a delicious full meal.

Per Serving

Calories: 200; Total Fat: 12g; Saturated Fat: 7g; Cholesterol: 78mg; Carbohydrates: 11g; Protein: 15g; Fiber: 2g; Sodium: 406mg

Parmesan Green Beans

PREP TIME: 15 MINUTES / **COOK TIME:** 7 MINUTES / **SERVES** 4 / 390°F

Green beans have always been one of my very favorite vegetables. They're even more delicious when coated with a bread crumb mixture and Parmesan cheese before cooking. To keep the calories low, serve these with a Greek yogurt–based dip rather than a heavy ranch dressing.

VEGETARIAN

Olive oil
1 cup whole-wheat panko bread crumbs
¼ cup grated Parmesan cheese
1 teaspoon garlic powder
½ teaspoon freshly ground black pepper
½ teaspoon salt
1 egg
1 pound fresh green beans, trimmed

1. Spray a fryer basket lightly with olive oil.

2. In a medium bowl, mix together the panko bread crumbs, Parmesan cheese, garlic powder, black pepper, and salt.

3. In a small, shallow bowl, whisk the egg.

4. Dip the green beans in the whisked egg and then coat in the panko bread crumb mixture.

5. Place the green beans in a single layer in the fryer basket. Spritz lightly with olive oil. You may need to cook more than one batch.

6. Air fry until light brown and crispy, 5 to 7 minutes.

Air Fry Like a Pro: If you have ever made green beans like these, you know that the coating can be very fragile, so be very gentle when removing the green beans from the air fryer.

Per Serving

Calories: 154; Total Fat: 3g; Saturated Fat: 2g; Cholesterol: 51mg; Carbohydrates:

23g; Protein: 10g; Fiber: 6g; Sodium: 455mg

Green Beans and New Potatoes

PREP TIME: 10 MINUTES / COOK TIME: 22 MINUTES / SERVES 6 / 390°F

New potatoes, also called baby potatoes, take less time to prepare than regular potatoes because you don't need to peel them (plus the skin is a great source of fiber, so why would you want to?). They also cook quickly due to their small size. Their creamy flavor is accentuated in the air fryer and contrasts nicely with the bright flavor of green beans in this easy-to-make recipe.

DAIRY-FREE

GLUTEN-FREE

VEGETARIAN

Olive oil
2 pounds new potatoes, each cut in half
2 teaspoons seasoned salt, divided
16 ounces fresh green beans, trimmed

1. Spray a fryer basket lightly with olive oil.

2. Add the new potatoes to the fryer basket and sprinkle with 1 teaspoon of seasoned salt. Lightly spray the potatoes with olive oil. You may need to cook them in batches.

3. Air fry for 10 minutes. Shake the basket and add the green beans and sprinkle with the remaining 1 teaspoon of seasoned salt. Lightly spray the potatoes and green beans with olive oil.

4. Air fry until the potatoes are fork tender and lightly browned, 8 to 12 more minutes. If you want the potatoes to be extra crispy, add a few minutes to the cook time and spray with a little extra olive oil.

Air Fry Like a Pro: Green beans cook much more quickly than potatoes. It is important to wait until the last half of the cooking process to add the green beans or they will overcook and may even burn.

Pair It With: I have always loved the flavors of green beans and new potatoes with Breaded Pork Cutlets.

Per Serving

Calories: 152; Total Fat: <1g; Saturated Fat: 0g; Cholesterol: 0mg; Carbohydrates: 33g; Protein: 6g; Fiber: 6g; Sodium: 511mg

Crunchy Hasselback Potatoes

PREP TIME: 15 MINUTES / **COOK TIME:** 50 MINUTES / **SERVES** 4 / 350°F

Originating from Sweden, Hasselback Potatoes make an eye-catching side dish. Potatoes are cut about three quarters of the way through and when cooked they fan out a bit, making the dish look like an accordion. It's a dramatic side dish to serve to guests or for a holiday meal, and one that doesn't require loads of butter or sour cream to make it tasty.

GLUTEN-FREE

VEGETARIAN

Olive oil
4 russet potatoes, peeled
Salt
Freshly ground black pepper
¼ cup grated Parmesan cheese

1. Spray a fryer basket lightly with olive oil.

2. Make thin parallel cuts into each potato, ⅛-inch to ¼-inch apart, stopping at about ½ of the way through. The potato needs to stay totally intact along the bottom.

3. Spray the potatoes with olive oil and use your hands or a silicone brush to completely coat the potatoes lightly in oil.

4. Place the potatoes, sliced side up, in the fryer basket in a single layer. Leave a little room between each potato. Sprinkle the potatoes lightly with salt and black pepper.

5. Air fry for 20 minutes. Reposition the potatoes and spritz lightly with more olive oil. Cook until the potatoes are fork tender and crispy and browned, another 20 to 30 minutes.

6. Sprinkle the potatoes with Parmesan cheese and serve.

Air Fry Like a Pro: The cook time will vary a lot depending on the size of the potatoes. Check for doneness at 20 minutes and continue cooking as needed.

Per Serving

Calories: 197; Total Fat: 2g; Saturated Fat: 1g; Cholesterol: 5mg; Carbohydrates: 39g; Protein: 7g; Fiber: 3g; Sodium: 127mg

Spicy Sweet Potatoes

PREP TIME: 10 MINUTES / **COOK TIME:** 15 MINUTES / **SERVES** 4 / 390°F

Sweet potatoes are much lower on the glycemic index than their white potato cousins, so they're better at controlling blood sugar and are less likely to cause weight gain. They are also high in vitamin A, which helps with immune function. In this recipe, their natural slight sweetness contrasts perfectly with the flavorful spices.

DAIRY-FREE

GLUTEN-FREE

VEGETARIAN

Olive oil
1½ teaspoon salt
1 teaspoon chili powder
1 teaspoon paprika
1 teaspoon onion powder
½ teaspoon ground cumin
½ teaspoon freshly ground black pepper
¼ teaspoon cayenne pepper
2 large sweet potatoes, peeled and cut into 1-inch pieces

1. Spray a fryer basket lightly with olive oil.

2. In a small bowl, combine the salt, chili powder, paprika, onion powder, cumin, black pepper, and cayenne pepper.

3. In a large bowl, add the sweet potato and spray lightly with olive oil. Add the seasoning mix and toss to coat.

4. Put the sweet potatoes in the fryer basket. Air fry until browned and slightly crispy, about 15 minutes, shaking the basket every 5 minutes and spraying lightly with olive oil each time. To make them extra crispy, cook for a few more minutes but watch closely to make sure they don't burn.

Air Fry Like a Pro: Cut the sweet potatoes into chunks that are approximately the same size, which will help them cook evenly. The more olive oil you spray on the sweet potatoes the crunchier they will end up, though be mindful as more oil will add calories. The sweet potatoes will be soft and delicious after about 10 minutes of air frying, but they won't be crispy.

Pair It With: These spicy sweet potatoes taste really great with <u>Chili-Lime Pork Loin</u>.

Per Serving

Calories: 88; Total Fat: <1g; Saturated Fat: 0g; Cholesterol: 0mg; Carbohydrates: 20g; Protein: 2g; Fiber: 4g; Sodium: 900mg

Portobello Pizzas

PREP TIME: 10 MINUTES / **COOK TIME:** 10 MINUTES / **SERVES** 4 / 350°F

Can you eat pizza while trying to lose weight? Only 25 calories each, these "pies" replace carb-heavy crusts with portobello mushrooms. Prep and cook times are very short, making them ideal for family movie night. Each person can top with their favorite healthy toppings.

Olive oil
4 large portobello mushroom caps, cleaned and stems removed
Garlic powder
8 tablespoons pizza sauce
16 slices turkey pepperoni
8 tablespoons mozzarella cheese

1. Spray a fryer basket lightly with olive oil.

2. Lightly spray the outside of the mushrooms with olive oil and sprinkle with a little garlic powder, to taste.

3. Turn the mushroom over and lightly spray the sides and top edges of the mushroom with olive oil and sprinkle with garlic powder, to taste.

4. Place the mushrooms in the fryer basket in a single layer with the top side down. Leave room between the mushrooms. You may need to cook them in batches.

5. Air fry for 5 minutes.

6. Spoon 2 tablespoons of pizza sauce on each mushroom. Top each with 4 slices of turkey pepperoni and sprinkle with 2 tablespoons of mozzarella cheese. Press the pepperoni and cheese down into the pizza sauce to help prevent it from flying around inside the air fryer.

7. Air fry until the cheese is melted and lightly browned on top, another 3 to 5 minutes.

Air Fry Like a Pro: Pushing the pepperoni down into the pizza sauce and mushroom will help keep the pizza toppings intact.

Per Serving

Calories: 103; Total Fat: 4g; Saturated Fat: 2g; Cholesterol: 14mg; Carbohydrates: 10g; Protein: 9g; Fiber: 2g; Sodium: 356mg

Creole Seasoned Okra

PREP TIME: 5 MINUTES / **COOK TIME:** 25 MINUTES / **SERVES** 4 / 350°F

Fried okra was a special treat my dad would make during the summer months when fresh varieties were plentiful. I love adapting dishes like this for the air fryer, with the goal of lightening up my childhood treats. In this case, I can use less oil and there's no need for breading to get that wonderful crispy crunch. I use frozen okra here, which is more readily available all year round.

DAIRY-FREE

GLUTEN-FREE

VEGETARIAN

1 teaspoon olive oil, plus more for spraying
12 ounces frozen sliced okra
1 to 2 teaspoons Creole seasoning

1. Spray a fryer basket lightly with olive oil.

2. In a medium bowl, toss the frozen okra with 1 teaspoon of olive oil and the Creole seasoning.

3. Place the okra into the fryer basket. You may need to cook them in batches.

4. Air fry until the okra is browned and crispy, 20 to 25 minutes, making sure to shake the basket and lightly spray with olive oil every 5 minutes.

Air Fry Like a Pro: The key to crunchy okra is to frequently shake the basket, which removes excess moisture. The okra will seem very wet during the first part of the cooking time but will eventually dry out and get crispy. Watch closely during the last 10 minutes of cooking. If you make this recipe with fresh okra, reduce air fry time to 10 to 15 minutes.

Per Serving

Calories: 31; Total Fat: 1g; Saturated Fat: <1g; Cholesterol: 0mg; Carbohydrates: 4g; Protein: 2g; Fiber: 2g; Sodium: 312mg

Easy Homemade Veggie Burger

PREP TIME: 15 MINUTES / **COOK TIME:** 26 MINUTES / **SERVES** 5 / 350°F

Plant-based burgers are a wonderful alternative to traditional beef burgers. And these are very easy to customize depending on the produce you have on hand. You'll need a total of about 2½ cups of chopped raw vegetables for this recipe. For example, if you don't care for mushrooms or carrots, simply substitute something like cauliflower, broccoli, or asparagus. The key is roasting the vegetables first to bring out their flavors.

DAIRY-FREE

VEGETARIAN

Olive oil
1 medium carrot, chopped very small
Salt
Freshly ground black pepper
8 ounces fresh mushrooms, stems removed, chopped very small
1 (15-ounce) can black beans, drained and rinsed
1 egg, beaten
2 tablespoons tomato paste
2 teaspoons minced garlic
½ teaspoon onion powder
¼ teaspoon salt
½ cup whole-wheat bread crumbs
5 whole-wheat hamburger buns

1. Spray a fryer basket lightly with olive oil.

2. Place the carrots in the fryer basket. Lightly spray with oil and season with salt and pepper.

3. Air fry for 8 minutes.

4. Add the mushrooms to the fryer basket with the carrots. Lightly spray with oil and season with a little more salt and pepper, if desired.

5. Air fry for 5 more minutes.

6. While the vegetables are roasting, spread the rinsed black beans out on a paper towel and dry them off. It is important to remove as much excess moisture as possible.

7. Place the black beans in a large bowl and mash them with a fork. If you like your veggie burger a little chunkier, leave some of the beans only partially mashed.

8. Add the egg, tomato paste, garlic, onion powder, salt, cooked carrots, and mushrooms to the bowl and mix together very well. Mash up the veggies with a fork if you prefer. Add the bread crumbs and stir to combine.

9. Form the mixture into 5 patties.

10. Add the patties to the fryer basket, leaving a little room between each patty. You may need to cook them in batches.

11. Air fry for 5 minutes. Flip the patties over and lightly spray with olive oil. Air fry for another 5 to 7 minutes.

12. Serve on whole-wheat buns.

Make It Lower Calorie: Skip the bun and wrap the patty in a lettuce leaf.

Per Serving

Calories: 272; Total Fat: 4g; Saturated Fat: 1g; Cholesterol: 37mg; Carbohydrates: 47g; Protein: 15g; Fiber: 11g; Sodium: 477mg

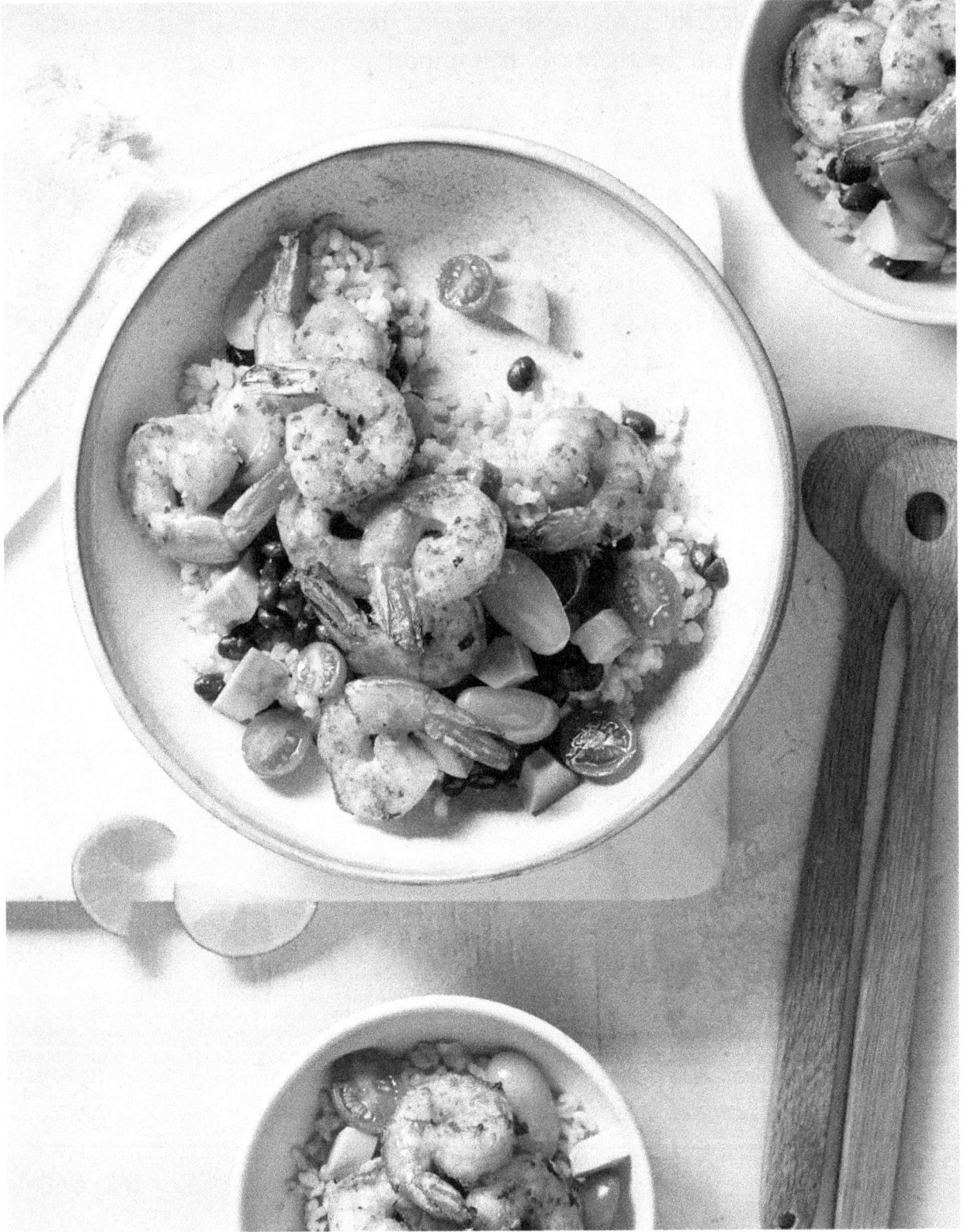

CHILI-LIME SHRIMP BOWL

CHAPTER 6

Fish and Seafood

Maryland Style Crab Cakes

Zesty Garlic Scallops

Spanish Garlic Shrimp

Blackened Shrimp Tacos

Chili-Lime Shrimp Bowl

Seasoned Breaded Shrimp

Country Shrimp "Boil"

Spicy Orange Shrimp

Seafood Spring Rolls

Lemon-Garlic Tilapia

Cajun Fish Tacos

Homemade Fish Sticks

Fish and Chips

Homestyle Catfish Strips

Quick Tuna Patty Sliders

Easy Marinated Salmon Fillets

Cajun Salmon Burger

Sesame-Glazed Salmon

Salmon Patty Bites

Crispy Breaded Calamari

Maryland-Style Crab Cakes

PREP TIME: 40 MINUTES / **COOK TIME:** 15 MINUTES / **SERVES** 6 / 360°F

While classic Maryland crab cakes are made using fresh blue crab, more readily available canned lump crab meat can help satisfy your crustacean cravings. Sweet and delicate, crab is not only delicious but also naturally low in fat and high in protein, which helps keep you full. Serve these with a reduced-fat tartar sauce.

DAIRY-FREE

4 (6-ounce) cans lump crab meat, drained
1 cup whole-wheat panko bread crumbs
1 cup chopped fresh parsley
4 cloves garlic, minced
4 teaspoons Dijon mustard
2 teaspoons Old Bay seasoning
2 large eggs, beaten
Olive oil

1. In a large bowl, mix together the crab meat, panko bread crumbs, parsley, garlic, Dijon mustard, and Old Bay seasoning. Add the eggs and stir to combine. Cover the bowl and refrigerate for 30 minutes.

2. Spray a fryer basket lightly with olive oil.

3. Form the mixture into 12 crab cakes.

4. Place the crab cakes in the fryer basket in a single layer. Spray the tops lightly with olive oil. You may need to cook them in batches.

5. Air fry for 6 to 8 minutes. Turn the crab cakes over, spray lightly with olive oil, and cook until golden brown, 4 to 7 more minutes.

Air Fry Like a Pro: Use a wide spatula when flipping over the crab cakes, which will keep them from falling apart.

Per Serving

Calories: 107; Total Fat: 2g; Saturated Fat: 1g; Cholesterol: 92mg; Carbohydrates: 11g; Protein: 11g; Fiber: 2g; Sodium: 458mg

Zesty Garlic Scallops

PREP TIME: 10 MINUTES / **COOK TIME:** 15 MINUTES / **SERVES** 4 / 400°F

With a slightly sweet taste and firm texture, scallops offer bountiful health benefits in addition to their low calories. They're high in protein, iron, vitamin B_{12}, and much more. I tend to favor smaller scallops at home, because they cook up quickly. Keep bags of them in your freezer for a quick, delicious dinner.

DAIRY-FREE

2 teaspoons olive oil, plus more for spraying
1 packet dry zesty Italian dressing mix
1 teaspoon minced garlic
16 ounces small scallops, thawed, patted dry

1. Spray a fryer basket lightly with olive oil.

2. In a large zip-top plastic bag, combine the olive oil, Italian dressing mix, and garlic.

3. Add the scallops, seal the zip-top bag, and coat the scallops in the seasoning mixture.

4. Place the scallops in the fryer basket and lightly spray with olive oil.

5. Air fry for 5 minutes, shake the basket, and cook until the scallops reach an internal temperature of 120°F, for 5 to 10 more minutes.

Pair It With: Make a full meal out of these scallops by adding them to a bowl of cooked quinoa and veggies.

Per Serving

Calories: 131; Total Fat: 3g; Saturated Fat: <1g; Cholesterol: 37mg; Carbohydrates: 5g; Protein: 19g; Fiber: 0g; Sodium: 823mg

Spanish Garlic Shrimp

PREP TIME: 10 MINUTES / **COOK TIME:** 15 MINUTES / **SERVES** 4 / 400°F

If you love bold flavors, this dish will become a favorite and you can adjust the crushed red pepper depending on how spicy you like it. In addition to being low calorie, shrimp is one of the best sources of iodine, an important ingredient for proper thyroid function and brain health.

DAIRY-FREE

GLUTEN-FREE

2 teaspoons olive oil plus more for spraying
2 teaspoons minced garlic
2 teaspoons lemon juice
½ to 1 teaspoon crushed red pepper
12 ounces medium cooked shrimp, thawed, and deveined, with tails on

1. Spray a fryer basket lightly with olive oil.

2. In a medium bowl, mix together the garlic, lemon juice, 2 teaspoons of olive oil, and crushed red pepper to make a marinade.

3. Add the shrimp and toss to coat in the marinade. Cover with plastic wrap and place the bowl in the refrigerator for 30 minutes.

4. Place the shrimp in the fryer basket. Air fry for 5 minutes. Shake the basket and cook until the shrimp are cooked through and nicely browned, an additional 5 to 10 minutes.

Pair It With: The garlicky flavor of this dish pairs nicely with the Cheesy Roasted Tomatoes.

Per Serving

Calories: 100; Total Fat: 3g; Saturated Fat: <1g; Cholesterol: 165mg; Carbohydrates: 1g; Protein: 17g; Fiber: <1g; Sodium: 468mg

Blackened Shrimp Tacos

PREP TIME: 10 MINUTES / **COOK TIME:** 15 MINUTES / **SERVES** 4 / 400°F

Blackening is a cooking technique that typically requires dipping a protein in melted butter and then coating in a combination of seasonings. By using a little olive oil instead of butter in the air fryer, you can enjoy this classic Cajun flavor without worrying about excessive calories from fat. You can buy blackened seasoning in the spice aisle at your local grocery store.

DAIRY-FREE

GLUTEN-FREE

1 teaspoon olive oil, plus more for spraying
12 ounces medium shrimp, deveined, tails off
1 to 2 teaspoons blackened seasoning
8 corn tortillas, warmed
1 (14-ounce) bag coleslaw mix
2 limes, cut in half

1. Spray a fryer basket lightly with olive oil.

2. Dry the shrimp with a paper towel to remove excess water.

3. In a medium bowl, toss the shrimp with 1 teaspoon of olive oil and blackened seasoning.

4. Place the shrimp in the fryer basket and cook for 5 minutes. Shake the basket, lightly spray with olive oil, and cook until the shrimp are cooked through and starting to brown, 5 to 10 more minutes.

5. Fill each tortilla with the coleslaw mix and top with the blackened shrimp. Squeeze fresh lime juice over top.

Pair It With: Serve the tacos with Crunchy Tex-Mex Tortilla Chips and some salsa on the side for a complete meal.

Per Serving (2 tacos)

Calories: 257; Total Fat: 4g; Saturated Fat: <1g; Cholesterol: 170mg; Carbohydrates: 33g; Protein: 25g; Fiber: 7g; Sodium: 552mg

Chili-Lime Shrimp Bowl

PREP TIME: 10 MINUTES / **COOK TIME:** 15 MINUTES / **SERVES** 4 / 400°F

The mild flavor of shrimp allows you to be creative with different seasoning combinations, and this chili-lime blend really helps them shine. When served over brown rice and chopped avocado, it's a dish that will keep you full long after mealtime.

DAIRY-FREE

GLUTEN-FREE

1 teaspoon olive oil, plus more for spraying
2 teaspoons lime juice
1 teaspoon honey
1 teaspoon minced garlic
1 teaspoon chili powder
Salt
12 ounces medium cooked shrimp, thawed, deveined, peeled
2 cups cooked brown rice
1 (15-ounce) can seasoned black beans, warmed
1 large avocado, chopped
1 cup sliced cherry tomatoes

1. Spray a fryer basket lightly with olive oil.

2. In a medium bowl, mix together the lime juice, 1 teaspoon of olive oil, honey, garlic, chili powder, and salt to make a marinade.

3. Add the shrimp and toss to coat evenly in the marinade.

4. Place the shrimp in the fryer basket. Air fry for 5 minutes. Shake the basket and cook until the shrimp are cooked through and starting to brown, an additional 5 to 10 minutes.

5. To assemble the bowls, spoon ¼ of the rice, black beans, avocado, and cherry tomatoes into each of four bowls. Top with the shrimp and serve.

Air Fry Like a Pro: Shaking the basket during the cook time allows you to check for doneness and avoid overcooked shrimp that sticks to the basket.

Per Serving

Calories: 412; Total Fat: 11g; Saturated Fat: 1g; Cholesterol: 170mg; Carbohydrates: 49g; Protein: 31g; Fiber: 10g; Sodium: 859mg

Seasoned Breaded Shrimp

PREP TIME: 15 MINUTES / **COOK TIME:** 15 MINUTES / **SERVES** 4 / 380°F

Breaded, fried shrimp are irresistible, but traditional deep-frying makes them a trans-fat nightmare. You can get them just as crisp and flavorful in the air-fryer using just a little oil and fiber-rich whole-wheat bread crumbs.

DAIRY-FREE

Olive oil
2 teaspoons Old Bay seasoning, divided
½ teaspoon garlic powder
½ teaspoon onion powder
1 pound large shrimp, deveined, with tails on
2 large eggs
½ cup whole-wheat panko bread crumbs

1. Spray a fryer basket lightly with olive oil.

2. In a medium bowl, mix together 1 teaspoon of Old Bay seasoning, garlic powder, and onion powder. Add the shrimp and toss with the seasoning mix to lightly coat.

3. In a separate small bowl whisk the eggs with 1 teaspoon water.

4. In a shallow bowl, mix together the remaining 1 teaspoon Old Bay seasoning and the panko bread crumbs.

5. Dip each shrimp in the egg mixture and dredge in the bread crumb mixture to evenly coat.

6. Place the shrimp in the fryer basket, in a single layer. Lightly spray the shrimp with oil. You many need to cook the shrimp in batches.

7. Air fry until the shrimp is cooked through and crispy, 10 to 15 minutes, shaking the basket at 5-minute intervals to redistribute and evenly cook.

Make it Gluten-Free: You can get gluten-free panko bread crumbs and they work just as well.

Per Serving

Calories: 183; Total Fat: 4g; Saturated Fat: 1g; Cholesterol: 263mg; Carbohydrates: 8g; Protein: 28g; Fiber: 1g; Sodium: 537mg

Country Shrimp "Boil"

PREP TIME: 10 MINUTES / **COOK TIME:** 20 MINUTES / **SERVES** 4 / 400°F

A Southern tradition, low country boils combine seafood and vegetables in a large pot of seasoned water. Although there is no actual boiling here, the recipe has all the same flavors with fewer calories.

DAIRY-FREE

GLUTEN-FREE

2 tablespoons olive oil, plus more for spraying
1 pound large shrimp, deveined, tail on
1 pound smoked turkey sausage, cut into thick slices
2 corn cobs, quartered
1 zucchini, cut into bite-sized pieces
1 red bell pepper, cut into chunks
1 tablespoon Old Bay seasoning

1. Spray the fryer basket lightly with olive oil.

2. In a large bowl, mix together the shrimp, turkey sausage, corn, zucchini, bell pepper, and Old Bay seasoning, and toss to coat with the spices. Add the 2 tablespoons of olive oil and toss again until evenly coated.

3. Spread the mixture in the fryer basket in a single layer. You will need to cook in batches.

4. Air fry until cooked through, 15 to 20 minutes, shaking the basket every 5 minutes for even cooking.

Make It Even Lower Calorie: Omit the turkey sausage and use 2 pounds of shrimp instead.

Per Serving

Calories: 436; Total Fat: 22g; Saturated Fat: 5g; Cholesterol: 230mg; Carbohydrates: 23g; Protein: 42g; Fiber: 3g; Sodium: 1,884mg

Spicy Orange Shrimp

PREP TIME: 40 MINUTES / **COOK TIME:** 15 MINUTES / **SERVES** 4 / 400°F

A combination of citrus, garlic, cayenne, and Old Bay seasoning gives this shrimp dish a uniquely bright flavor. Even with just a half-hour of marinating, the flavors really soak in, and the shrimp comes out of the fryer crispy and delicious.

DAIRY-FREE

GLUTEN-FREE

Olive oil
⅓ cup orange juice
3 teaspoons minced garlic
1 teaspoon Old Bay seasoning
¼ to ½ teaspoon cayenne pepper
1 pound medium shrimp, thawed, deveined, peeled, with tails off

1. Spray a fryer basket lightly with olive oil.

2. In a medium bowl, combine the orange juice, garlic, Old Bay seasoning, and cayenne pepper.

3. Dry the shrimp with paper towels to remove excess water.

4. Add the shrimp to the marinade and stir to evenly coat. Cover with plastic wrap and place in the refrigerator for 30 minutes so the shrimp can soak up the marinade.

5. Place the shrimp into the fryer basket. Air fry for 5 minutes. Shake the basket and lightly spray with olive oil. Cook until the shrimp are opaque and crisp, 5 to 10 more minutes.

Pair It With: The sweetness of Crispy Breaded Bell Pepper Strips provides a nice complement to this dish.

Per Serving

Calories: 146; Total Fat: 2g; Saturated Fat: 0g; Cholesterol: 227mg; Carbohydrates: 3g; Protein: 28g; Fiber: <1g; Sodium: 785mg

Seafood Spring Rolls

PREP TIME: 10 MINUTES / **COOK TIME:** 22 MINUTES / **SERVES** 4 / 370°F

I have tried to bake spring rolls in the oven but have never been satisfied with the results. The air fryer can cook them to the requisite crispiness without dunking them in oil.

DAIRY-FREE

Olive oil
2 teaspoon minced garlic
2 cups finely sliced cabbage
1 cup matchstick cut carrots
2 (4-ounce) cans tiny shrimp, drained
4 teaspoons soy sauce
Salt
Freshly ground black pepper
16 square spring roll wrappers

1. Spray a fryer basket lightly with olive oil. Spray a medium sauté pan with olive oil.

2. Add the garlic to the sauté pan and cook over medium heat until fragrant, 30 to 45 seconds. Add the cabbage and carrots and sauté until the vegetables are slightly tender, about 5 minutes.

3. Add the shrimp and soy sauce and season with salt and pepper, then stir to combine. Sauté until the moisture has evaporated, 2 more minutes. Set aside to cool.

4. Place a spring roll wrapper on a work surface so it looks like a diamond. Place 1 tablespoon of the shrimp mixture on the lower end of the wrapper.

5. Roll the wrapper away from you halfway, then fold in the right and left sides, like an envelope. Continue to roll to the very end, using a little water to seal the edge. Repeat with the remaining wrappers and filling.

6. Place the spring rolls in the fryer basket in a single layer, leaving room between each roll. Lightly spray with olive oil. You may need to cook them

in batches.

7. Air fry for 5 minutes. Turn the rolls over, lightly spray with olive oil, and cook until heated through and the rolls start to brown, 5 to 10 more minutes.

Per Serving

Calories: 159; Total Fat: 1g; Saturated Fat: <1g; Cholesterol: 118mg; Carbohydrates: 24g; Protein: 14g; Fiber: 2g; Sodium: 941mg

Lemon-Garlic Tilapia

PREP TIME: 10 MINUTES / **COOK TIME:** 15 MINUTES / **SERVES** 4 / 380°F

Tilapia is a white freshwater fish with a mild flavor that is a great base for a variety of recipes. It is a gateway fish for anyone hesitant about eating seafood. It is also readily available as skinless, boneless fillets, fresh or frozen.

DAIRY-FREE

GLUTEN-FREE

1 tablespoon lemon juice
1 tablespoon olive oil
1 teaspoon minced garlic
½ teaspoon chili powder
4 (5 to 6 ounce) tilapia fillets

1. Line a fryer basket with perforated air fryer liners.

2. In a large, shallow bowl, mix together the lemon juice, olive oil, garlic, and chili powder to make a marinade. Place the tilapia fillets in the bowl and coat evenly.

3. Place the fillets in the basket in a single layer, leaving space between each fillet. You may need to cook in more than one batch.

4. Air fry until the fish is cooked and flakes easily with a fork, 10 to 15 minutes.

Air Fry Like a Pro: The cooking time will depend on the thickness of the fillets. It's best not to flip the fillets over because they are very fragile and are likely to break. You can easily buy perforated air fryer liners online. Keep them on hand for recipes like this.

Per Serving

Calories: 169; Total Fat: 6g; Saturated Fat: 1g; Cholesterol: 73mg; Carbohydrates: 1g; Protein: 29g; Fiber: 0g; Sodium: 76mg

Cajun Fish Tacos

PREP TIME: 10 MINUTES / **COOK TIME:** 15 MINUTES / **SERVES** 6 / 380°F

Tacos made with soft corn tortillas are generally a healthy option, but they become calorie-laden if too many fattening toppings are added. This recipe uses tilapia lightly coated in avocado oil (a "good" fat), vitamin-rich cabbage, the festive flavors of Cajun seasoning, and fresh lime juice.

DAIRY-FREE

GLUTEN-FREE

2 teaspoons avocado oil
1 tablespoon Cajun seasoning
4 (5 to 6 ounce) tilapia fillets
1 (14-ounce) package coleslaw mix
12 corn tortillas
2 limes, cut into wedges

1. Line a fryer basket with a perforated air fryer liner.

2. In a medium, shallow bowl mix together the avocado oil and the Cajun seasoning to make a marinade. Add the tilapia fillets and coat evenly.

3. Place the fillets in the basket in a single layer, leaving room between each fillet. You may need to cook in batches.

4. Air fry until the fish is cooked and easily flakes with a fork, 10 to 15 minutes.

5. Assemble the tacos by placing some of the coleslaw mix in each tortilla. Add ⅓ of a tilapia fillet to each tortilla. Squeeze some lime juice over the top of each taco and serve.

Pair It With: Creole Seasoned Okra is a perfect accompaniment to the Cajun flavors of these tacos.

Per Serving

Calories: 242; Total Fat: 5g; Saturated Fat: 1g; Cholesterol: 48mg; Carbohydrates: 30g; Protein: 23g; Fiber: 6g; Sodium: 356mg

Homemade Fish Sticks

PREP TIME: 15 MINUTES / **COOK TIME:** 15 MINUTES / **SERVES** 4 / 400°F

Frozen fish sticks were one of my favorite meals when I was a kid. As an adult, they bring back pleasant nostalgic memories, but now I make them using fresh fish and coat them in fiber-rich whole-wheat flour. This healthier air-fried rendition can be made with any firm white fish such as cod, pollack, or tilapia. Your kids will love them.

DAIRY-FREE

Olive oil
4 fish fillets (cod, tilapia or pollock)
½ cup whole-wheat flour
1 teaspoon seasoned salt
2 eggs
1½ cups whole-wheat panko bread crumbs
½ tablespoon dried parsley flakes

1. Spray a fryer basket lightly with olive oil.

2. Cut the fish fillets lengthwise into "sticks."

3. In a shallow bowl, mix together the whole-wheat flour and seasoned salt.

4. In a small bowl whisk the eggs with 1 teaspoon of water.

5. In another shallow bowl, mix together the panko bread crumbs and parsley flakes.

6. Coat each fish stick in the seasoned flour, then in the egg mixture, and dredge them in the panko bread crumbs.

7. Place the fish sticks in the fryer basket in a single layer and lightly spray the fish sticks with olive oil. You may need to cook them in batches.

8. Air fry for 5 to 8 minutes. Flip the fish sticks over and lightly spray with the olive oil. Cook until golden brown and crispy, 5 to 7 more minutes.

Air Fry Like a Pro: You can skip the parchment paper for these, as the breading will keep them from sticking.

Per Serving

Calories: 302; Total Fat: 5g; Saturated Fat: 2g; Cholesterol: 151mg; Carbohydrates: 32g; Protein: 33g; Fiber: 5g; Sodium: 511mg

Fish and Chips

PREP TIME: 25 MINUTES / **COOK TIME:** 35 MINUTES / **SERVES** 4 / 400°F

Fish and chips are traditionally loaded with grease and fat. A typical serving usually has 25 or more grams of fat. But this recipe dramatically reduces the fat content so you can enjoy this British classic without forgoing your weight-loss goal—and it's authentic enough to wrap in your daily newspaper.

DAIRY-FREE

For the chips
1 tablespoon olive oil, plus more for spraying
2 large russet potatoes, scrubbed
1 teaspoon salt
½ teaspoon freshly ground black pepper

For the fish
Olive oil
4 (4-ounce) cod fillets
1½ teaspoons salt, divided plus more as needed
1½ teaspoons black pepper, divided, plus more as needed
½ cup whole-wheat flour
2 eggs
1½ cups whole-wheat panko bread crumbs
¼ teaspoon cayenne pepper

To make the chips

1. Spray a fryer basket lightly with olive oil.

2. Cut the potatoes lengthwise into ½-inch-thick slices and then into ½-inch-thick fries.

3. In a large bowl, mix together the oil, salt, and pepper and toss with the potatoes to coat.

4. Place the potatoes in a single layer in the fryer basket. You may need to cook them in batches.

5. Air fry for 5 minutes. Shake the basket and cook until the potatoes are

lightly browned and crisp, 5 to 10 more minutes. Set aside and keep warm.

To make the fish

6. Spray the fryer basket with olive oil.

7. Season the fillets with salt and black pepper.

8. In a shallow bowl, mix together the whole-wheat flour, ½ teaspoon of salt, and ½ teaspoon of black pepper.

9. In a second bowl, whisk together the eggs, 1 teaspoon of water, and a pinch of salt and pepper.

10. In another shallow bowl, combine the panko bread crumbs, cayenne pepper, and remaining 1 teaspoon of salt and 1 teaspoon of black pepper.

11. Coat each fillet in the seasoned flour, then coat with the egg, and dredge in the panko bread crumb mixture.

12. Place the fillets in the fryer basket in a single layer. Lightly spray the fish with olive oil. You may need to cook them in batches.

13. Air fry for 8 to 10 minutes. Turn the fillets over and lightly spray with olive oil. Cook until golden brown and crispy, 5 to 10 more minutes.

Make It Lower Calorie: If you like to serve fish and chips with tartar sauce, try making your own healthier version by using Greek yogurt or nonfat sour cream as a base with your favorite recipe.

Per Serving

Calories: 370; Total Fat: 6g; Saturated Fat: 1g; Cholesterol: 93mg; Carbohydrates: 66g; Protein: 14g; Fiber: 8g; Sodium: 1,524mg

Homestyle Catfish Strips

PREP TIME: 1 HOUR 15 MINUTES / **COOK TIME:** 20 MINUTES / **SERVES** 4 / 400°F

Catfish is a great source of omega-3 fatty acid, which has been shown to help prevent heart attacks and lower blood sugar levels. There are many ways to prepare catfish, but frying is one of the most common preparations. This air-fryer recipe gets them just as crunchy without requiring a swim in trans fat–loaded oil.

GLUTEN-FREE

1 cup buttermilk
5 catfish fillets, cut into 1½-inch strips
Olive oil
1 cup cornmeal
1 tablespoon Creole, Cajun, or Old Bay seasoning

1. Pour the buttermilk into a shallow baking dish. Place the catfish in the dish and refrigerate for at least 1 hour to help remove any fishy taste.

2. Spray a fryer basket lightly with olive oil.

3. In a shallow bowl, combine cornmeal and Creole seasoning.

4. Shake any excess buttermilk off the catfish. Place each strip in the cornmeal mixture and coat completely. Press the cornmeal into the catfish gently to help it stick.

5. Place the strips in the fryer basket in a single layer. Lightly spray the catfish with olive oil. You may need to cook the catfish in more than one batch.

6. Air fry for 8 minutes. Turn the catfish strips over and lightly spray with olive oil. Cook until golden brown and crispy, 8 to 10 more minutes.

Pair It With: Make this a bayou-worthy meal by serving it with Spicy Corn on the Cob.

Per Serving

Calories: 260; Total Fat: 4g; Saturated Fat: 1g; Cholesterol: 84mg; Carbohydrates: 26g; Protein: 30g; Fiber: 2g; Sodium: 1,100mg

Quick Tuna Patty Sliders

PREP TIME: 15 MINUTES / **COOK TIME:** 15 MINUTES / **SERVES** 4 / 350°F

Canned tuna is an inexpensive, healthy protein to keep in the pantry for a quick lunch or dinner, and this recipe is a nice change from typical tuna sandwiches. The sriracha and black pepper bring a little dash of heat and flavor to the patties, and whole-wheat buns help keep your carbs on the healthy side.

Olive oil
3 (5-ounce) cans tuna, packed in water
⅔ cup whole-wheat panko bread crumbs
⅓ cup shredded Parmesan cheese
1 tablespoon sriracha
¾ teaspoon black pepper
10 whole-wheat slider buns

1. Spray a fryer basket lightly with olive oil.

2. In a medium bowl combine the tuna, bread crumbs, Parmesan cheese, sriracha, and black pepper and stir to combine.

3. Form the mixture into 10 patties.

4. Place the patties in the fryer basket in a single layer. Spray the patties lightly with olive oil. You may need to cook them in batches.

5. Air fry for 6 to 8 minutes. Turn the patties over and lightly spray with olive oil. Cook until golden brown and crisp, another 4 to 7 more minutes.

Make It Gluten-Free: Use gluten-free bread crumbs and buns.

Pair It With: Parmesan Green Beans make a healthy alternative to fries.

Per Serving

Calories: 401; Total Fat: 7g; Saturated Fat: 1g; Cholesterol: 37mg; Carbohydrates: 55g; Protein: 30g; Fiber: 9g; Sodium: 976mg

Easy Marinated Salmon Fillets

PREP TIME: 10 MINUTES, PLUS 1 HOUR TO MARINATE / **COOK TIME:** 20 MINUTES / **SERVES** 4 / 370°F

On a trip to Alaska, I had the memorable experience of seeing salmon swimming upstream to spawn. We finished the day with a meal made with the freshest salmon I have ever had, which gave me a whole new appreciation for this hearty, versatile seafood that's rich in omega-3 fatty acids, B vitamins, and potassium. Salmon is higher in calories than other fish but it's still lower than other proteins.

DAIRY-FREE

GLUTEN-FREE

1 tablespoon olive oil, plus more for spraying
¼ cup soy sauce
¼ cup rice wine vinegar
1 tablespoon brown sugar
1 teaspoon mustard powder
1 teaspoon ground ginger
½ teaspoon freshly ground black pepper
½ teaspoon minced garlic
4 (6 ounce) salmon fillets, skin-on

1. Spray a fryer basket lightly with olive oil.

2. In a small bowl combine the soy sauce, rice wine vinegar, brown sugar, 1 tablespoon of olive oil, mustard powder, ginger, black pepper, and garlic to make a marinade.

3. Place the fillets in a shallow baking dish and pour the marinade over them. Cover the baking dish and marinate for at least 1 hour in the refrigerator, turning the fillets occasionally to keep them coated in the marinade.

4. Shake off as much marinade as possible from the fillets and place them, skin side down, in the fryer basket in a single layer. You may need to cook the fillets in batches.

5. Air fry for 10 to 15 minutes for medium-rare to medium done salmon or 15 to 20 minutes for well done. The minimum internal temperature should be 145°F at the thickest part of the fillet.

Air Fry Like a Pro: The cooking time will vary based on the size and thickness of the salmon fillet. Using skin-on salmon fillets is convenient because the skin will not stick to the basket. If you prefer to use skinless fillets, line the fryer basket with perforated parchment paper to prevent sticking.

Per Serving

Calories: 260; Total Fat: 10g; Saturated Fat: 2g; Cholesterol: 128mg; Carbohydrates: 5g; Protein: 36g; Fiber: <1g; Sodium: 982mg

Cajun Salmon Burgers

PREP TIME: 40 MINUTES / **COOK TIME:** 15 MINUTES / **SERVES** 4 / 360°F

Salmon burgers are similar to salmon croquettes, which originated in France. These are a great alternative to regular beef burgers because they are very flavorful, especially with a little Cajun seasoning and dry mustard; they also have a much lower calorie count. This recipe uses canned salmon, so it's an easy last-minute meal.

DAIRY-FREE

Olive oil
4 (5-ounce) cans pink salmon in water, any skin and bones removed, drained
2 eggs, beaten
1 cup whole-wheat bread crumbs
4 tablespoons light mayonnaise
2 teaspoons Cajun seasoning
2 teaspoons dry mustard
4 whole-wheat buns

1. Spray a fryer basket lightly with olive oil.

2. In a medium bowl, mix together the salmon, egg, bread crumbs, mayonnaise, Cajun seasoning, and dry mustard. Cover with plastic wrap and refrigerate for 30 minutes.

3. Shape the mixture into four ½-inch-thick patties about the same size as the buns.

4. Place the salmon patties in the fryer basket in a single layer and lightly spray the tops with olive oil. You may need to cook them in batches.

5. Air fry for 6 to 8 minutes. Turn the patties over and lightly spray with olive oil. Cook until crispy on the outside, 4 to 7 more minutes.

6. Serve on whole-wheat buns.

Pair It With: Carrot Chips make a nice side dish with these burgers.

Per Serving

Calories: 391; Total Fat: 12g; Saturated Fat: 1g; Cholesterol: 138mg; Carbohydrates: 39g; Protein: 32g; Fiber: 6g; Sodium: 1,204mg

Sesame-Glazed Salmon

PREP TIME: 1 HOUR 10 MINUTES / **COOK TIME:** 16 MINUTES / **SERVES** 4 / 370°F TO 400°F

The ginger in this marinade not only packs a flavor punch but is also an appetite suppressant. Easy enough for a weeknight dinner, this dish also feels elevated enough to serve to guests.

DAIRY-FREE

GLUTEN-FREE

3 tablespoons soy sauce
1 tablespoon rice wine or dry sherry
1 tablespoon brown sugar
1 tablespoon toasted sesame oil
1 teaspoon minced garlic
¼ teaspoon minced ginger
4 (6 ounce) salmon fillets, skin-on
Olive oil
½ tablespoon sesame seeds

1. In a small bowl, mix together the soy sauce, rice wine, brown sugar, toasted sesame oil, garlic, and ginger.

2. Place the salmon in a shallow baking dish and pour the marinade over the fillets. Cover and refrigerate for at least 1 hour, turning the fillets occasionally to coat in the marinade.

3. Spray a fryer basket lightly with olive oil.

4. Shake off as much marinade as possible and place the fillets, skin side down, in the fryer basket in a single layer. Reserve the marinade. You may need to cook them in batches.

5. Air fry for 8 to 10 minutes. Brush the tops of the salmon fillets with the reserved marinade and sprinkle with sesame seeds.

6. Increase the fryer temperature to 400°F and cook for 2 to 5 more minutes for medium, 1 to 3 minutes for medium rare, or 4 to 6 minutes for well

done.

Pair It With: Start your meal off with some <u>Garlic Edamame</u> for the perfect precursor to the salmon.

Per Serving

Calories: 280; Total Fat: 11g; Saturated Fat: 2g; Cholesterol: 128mg; Carbohydrates: 8g; Protein: 36g; Fiber: <1g; Sodium: 805mg

Salmon Patty Bites

PREP TIME: 15 MINUTES / **COOK TIME:** 15 MINUTES / **SERVES** 4 / 360°F

Getting kids to try salmon may be a challenge if you have picky eaters in your household. These meatball-sized bites may just hook them—and kids will love helping you make them using a cookie scoop. Whole-wheat panko bread crumbs add a hearty crunch, while red bell pepper adds just a touch of sweetness.

DAIRY-FREE

Olive oil
4 (5-ounce) cans pink salmon, skinless, boneless in water, drained
2 eggs, beaten
1 cup whole-wheat panko bread crumbs
4 tablespoons finely minced red bell pepper
2 tablespoons parsley flakes
2 teaspoons Old Bay seasoning

1. Spray a fryer basket lightly with olive oil.

2. In a medium bowl, mix together the salmon, eggs, panko bread crumbs, red bell pepper, parsley flakes, and Old Bay seasoning.

3. Using a small cookie scoop, form the mixture into 20 balls.

4. Place the salmon bites in the fryer basket in a single layer and spray lightly with olive oil. You may need to cook them in batches.

5. Air fry until crispy for 10 to 15 minutes, shaking the basket a couple of times for even cooking.

Pair It With: Serve with Simple Roasted Cauliflower, a hearty, filling source of fiber and a multitude of vitamins.

Per Serving

Calories: 230; Total Fat: 6g; Saturated Fat: 1g; Cholesterol: 133mg; Carbohydrates: 15g; Protein: 26g; Fiber: 2g; Sodium: 942mg

Crispy Breaded Calamari

PREP TIME: 15 MINUTES / **COOK TIME:** 15 MINUTES / **SERVES** 4 / 380°F

A classic (and high-calorie) Italian appetizer, calamari are easy to make in the air fryer without using all the oil necessary for deep-frying. Whole-wheat flour and bread crumbs make this dish even more healthy, and they're delicious dipped in a low-sugar marinara or cocktail sauce.

DAIRY-FREE

Olive oil
1 pound fresh calamari tubes, rinsed and patted dry
½ teaspoon salt, plus more as needed
½ teaspoon pepper, plus more as needed
1 cup whole-wheat flour
3 eggs
1 cup whole-wheat bread crumbs
2 teaspoons dried parsley

1. Spray a fryer basket lightly with olive oil.

2. Cut the calamari into ¼-inch rings. Season them with salt and black pepper.

3. In a shallow bowl, combine the whole-wheat flour and ½ teaspoon of salt and ½ teaspoon of black pepper.

4. In a small bowl, whisk the eggs with 1 teaspoon of water.

5. In another shallow bowl, combine the bread crumbs and parsley.

6. Coat the calamari in the flour mixture, coat in the egg, and dredge in the bread crumbs to coat.

7. Place the calamari in the fryer basket in a single layer. Spray the calamari lightly with olive oil. You may need to cook the calamari in batches.

8. Air fry until crispy and lightly browned, 10 to 15 minutes, shaking the basket a few times during cooking to redistribute and evenly cook.

Air Fry Like a Pro: You can use frozen calamari, but be sure to thaw them and pat them dry before breading.

Per Serving

Calories: 337; Total Fat: 6g; Saturated Fat: 1g; Cholesterol: 400mg; Carbohydrates: 40g; Protein: 29g; Fiber: 6g; Sodium: 418mg

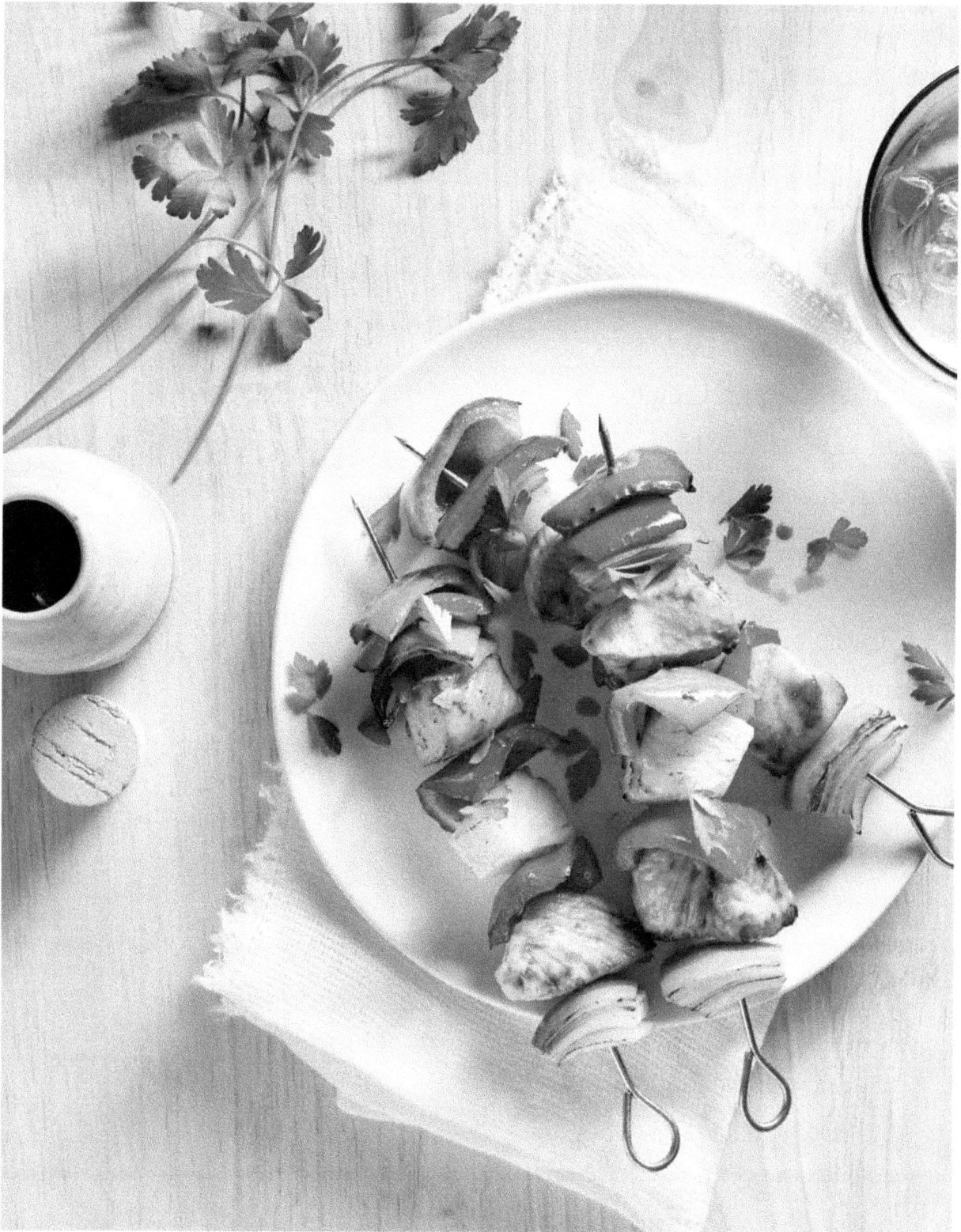

HAWAIIAN PINEAPPLE CHICKEN KEBABS

CHAPTER 7

Poultry

Cajun Chicken Kebabs

Hawaiian Pineapple Chicken Kebabs

Sesame Chicken Tenders

Teriyaki Chicken Bowls

Buffalo Chicken Taquitos

Jerk Chicken Wraps

Spinach and Feta Chicken Meatballs

Breaded Homestyle Chicken Strips

Black Pepper Chicken

Mexican Sheet Pan Dinner

Parmesan-Lemon Chicken

Italian Chicken and Veggies

Whole Roasted Chicken

Creole Cornish Hens

Sweet and Spicy Turkey Meatballs

Stuffed Bell Peppers

Hoisin Turkey Burgers

Easy Turkey Tenderloins

Apricot-Glazed Turkey Tenderloin

Herb-Roasted Turkey Breast

Cajun Chicken Kebabs

PREP TIME: 20 MINUTES / **COOK TIME:** 20 MINUTES / **SERVES** 6 / 350°F

Kebabs are delicious and fun to make with the whole family. The air fryer creates a delightful caramelized effect, without the hassle of having to fire up the grill. You will need skewers that fit into the air fryer.

DAIRY-FREE

GLUTEN-FREE

Olive oil
1½ pounds boneless, skinless chicken breasts, cut into bite-sized chunks
1½ tablespoons Cajun seasoning, divided
1 medium red bell pepper, cut into big chunks
1 medium green bell pepper, cut into big chunks
1 medium onion, cut into big chunks

1. Spray a fryer basket lightly with olive oil.

2. In a large bowl, toss the chicken with 1 tablespoon of Cajun seasoning, and spray with olive oil to coat.

3. In a separate, large bowl, toss the bell peppers and onion with the remaining ½ tablespoon of Cajun seasoning, and spray with olive oil to coat.

4. If using wooden skewers, soak them in water for at least 30 minutes before using.

5. Thread the chicken and vegetables onto the skewers, alternating with chicken, then vegetable.

6. Place the skewers in the fryer basket in a single layer. You may need to cook them in batches.

7. Air fry for 10 minutes. Flip the skewers over and lightly spray with olive oil. Air fry until the chicken has an internal temperature of at least 165°F, another 5 to 10 minutes.

Per Serving

Calories: 128; Total Fat: 3g; Saturated Fat: 1g; Cholesterol: 65mg; Carbohydrates: 4g; Protein: 24g; Fiber: 1g; Sodium: 766mg

Hawaiian Pineapple Chicken Kebabs

PREP TIME: 15 MINUTES, PLUS 1 TO 2 HOURS TO MARINATE / COOK TIME: 20 MINUTES / SERVES 6 / 350°F

The flavors of the Hawaiian islands shine through in these healthy, easy kebabs. Pineapple caramelizes in the air fryer, creating a crunchy, sweet treat that pairs perfectly with the mild chicken flavor. You'll even get an extra dose of vitamin C from the juice. You will need skewers that fit into the air fryer and if they are wooden, soak them in water for at least 30 minutes before using. Change this recipe up by adding things like red onion or cherry tomatoes.

DAIRY-FREE

Olive oil
3 tablespoons soy sauce
1 (15-ounce) can pineapple chunks, 2 tablespoons of the juice reserved
1 tablespoon sesame oil
¼ teaspoon ground ginger
¼ teaspoon garlic powder
1½ pounds boneless, skinless chicken breasts, cut into 1-inch chunks
2 large bell peppers, cut into 1-inch chunks

1. Spray a fryer basket lightly with olive oil.

2. In a large bowl, mix together the soy sauce, the reserved pineapple juice, sesame oil, ginger, and garlic powder. Add the chicken, bell peppers, and pineapple chunks and toss to coat.

3. Cover the bowl and refrigerate for at least 1 hour and up to 2 hours.

4. If using wooden skewers, soak the skewers in water for at least 30 minutes.

5. Thread the chicken, bell peppers, and pineapple onto the skewers, alternating with chicken, vegetable, and fruit. Place the skewers in the fryer basket in a single layer. Lightly spray the skewers with olive oil. You may need to cook the kebabs in batches.

6. Air fry for 10 minutes. Turn the skewers over, lightly spray with olive oil, and cook until the chicken is nicely browned and the veggies are starting to

char on the edges, an additional 5 to 10 minutes.

Per Serving

Calories: 190; Total Fat: 5g; Saturated Fat: 1g; Cholesterol: 65mg; Carbohydrates: 14g; Protein: 24g; Fiber: 2g; Sodium: 632mg

Sesame Chicken Tenders

PREP TIME: 5 MINUTES, PLUS 2 HOURS TO MARINATE / **COOK TIME:** 15 MINUTES / **SERVES** 4 / 375°F

Honey has been used both as a food and as a medicine since ancient times because it contains many antioxidants. Locally sourced honey can even help with seasonal allergies. Although honey is a naturally occurring sugar that is high in calories, using small quantities in sauces and marinades is a great natural way to add flavor. You will need skewers that fit into the air fryer and if they are wooden, soak them in water for at least 30 minutes before using.

DAIRY-FREE

Olive oil
¼ cup soy sauce
2 tablespoons white vinegar
1 tablespoon honey
1 tablespoon toasted sesame oil
1 tablespoon lime juice
1 teaspoon ground ginger
1 pound boneless skinless, chicken tenderloins
2 teaspoon toasted sesame seeds

1. Spray a fryer basket lightly with olive oil.

2. In a large zip-top plastic bag, combine the soy sauce, white vinegar, honey, sesame oil, lime juice, and ginger to make a marinade.

3. Add the chicken tenderloins to the bag, seal, and marinate the chicken in the refrigerator for at least 2 hours or overnight.

4. If using wooden skewers, soak them in water for at least 30 minutes before using.

5. Thread 1 chicken tenderloin onto each skewer. Sprinkle with sesame seeds. Reserve the marinade.

6. Place the skewers in the fryer basket in a single layer. You may need to cook the chicken in batches.

7. Air fry for 6 minutes. Flip the chicken over, baste with more marinade, and cook until crispy, an additional 5 to 8 minutes.

Pair It With: Spiced Balsamic Asparagus is a nice side dish for this meal.

Per Serving

Calories: 176; Total Fat: 7g; Saturated Fat: 1g; Cholesterol: 65mg; Carbohydrates: 6g; Protein: 24g; Fiber: <1g; Sodium: 1,079mg

Teriyaki Chicken Bowls

PREP TIME: 5 MINUTES, PLUS UP TO 30 MINUTES TO MARINATE / **COOK TIME:** 15 MINUTES / **SERVES** 4 / 375°F

The sweet and tangy flavor of teriyaki marinade is magical when combined with lean chicken tenderloins. This recipe calls for honey rather than a store-bought teriyaki marinade that tends to be high in sugar (and preservatives). Brown rice and steamed vegetables round out your bowl for a satisfying quick lunch or dinner.

DAIRY-FREE

Olive oil
⅓ cup soy sauce
⅓ cup honey
3 tablespoons white vinegar
1½ teaspoons dried thyme
1½ teaspoons paprika
1 teaspoon ground black pepper
½ teaspoon cayenne pepper
½ teaspoon ground allspice
1 pound boneless, skinless chicken tenderloins
2 cups cooked brown rice
2 cups steamed broccoli florets

1. Spray a fryer basket lightly with olive oil.

2. In a large bowl, mix together the soy sauce, honey, white vinegar, thyme, paprika, black pepper, cayenne pepper, and allspice to make a marinade.

3. Add the tenderloins to the marinade and stir to coat. Cover and refrigerate for 30 minutes.

4. Place the chicken in the fryer basket in a single layer. You may need to cook the chicken in batches. Reserve the marinade.

5. Air fry for 6 minutes. Turn the chicken over and brush with some of the remaining marinade. Cook until chicken reaches an internal temperature of at least 165°F, an additional 5 to 7 minutes.

6. To assemble the bowls, place ½ cup of brown rice, ½ cup of steamed broccoli, and 2 chicken tenderloins into each bowl and serve.

Make It Gluten-Free: Use a gluten-free soy sauce.

Per Serving

Calories: 335; Total Fat: 4g; Saturated Fat: 1g; Cholesterol: 65mg; Carbohydrates: 50g; Protein: 27g; Fiber: 4g; Sodium: 1,379mg

Buffalo Chicken Taquitos

PREP TIME: 15 MINUTES / **COOK TIME:** 10 MINUTES / **SERVES** 6 / 360°F

The flavor of Buffalo wings combined with everyone's favorite Mexican-style snack equals absolutely delicious. Fat-free cream cheese keeps the calories to a minimum, while the low-carb tortillas crisp up nicely in the air fryer. If you want to dip these taquitos in something, go for low-fat ranch dressing, but they taste great on their own as well.

Olive oil
8 ounces fat-free cream cheese, softened
⅛ cup Buffalo sauce
2 cups shredded cooked chicken
12 (7-inch) low-carb flour tortillas

1. Spray a fryer basket lightly with olive oil.

2. In a large bowl, mix together the cream cheese and Buffalo sauce until well-combined. Add the chicken and stir until combined.

3. Place the tortillas on a clean workspace. Spoon 2 to 3 tablespoons of the chicken mixture in a thin line down the center of each tortilla. Roll up the tortillas.

4. Place the tortillas in the fryer basket, seam side down. Spray each tortilla lightly with olive oil. You may need to cook the taquitos in batches.

5. Air fry until golden brown, 5 to 10 minutes.

Air Fry Like a Pro: Buy a cooked rotisserie chicken at your local grocery store, which is a great timesaver when making this recipe, plus you'll have leftovers to use in other meals.

Per Serving

Calories: 286; Total Fat: 8g; Saturated Fat: 3g; Cholesterol: 38mg; Carbohydrates: 25g; Protein: 28g; Fiber: 12g; Sodium: 919mg

Jerk Chicken Wraps

PREP TIME: 1 HOUR 10 MINUTES / **COOK TIME:** 15 MINUTES / **SERVES** 4 / 375°F

Keeping the pantry stocked with seasoning blends and marinades is a convenient way to get an appetizing meal on the table quickly. Jerk marinade is a delectable blend of sweet and salty with lots of spice along the way. It's a wonderful complement to the fresh fruits and vegetables in these wraps.

DAIRY-FREE

1 pound boneless, skinless chicken tenderloins
1 cup jerk marinade
Olive oil
4 large low-carb tortillas
1 cup julienned carrots
1 cup peeled cucumber ribbons
1 cup shredded lettuce
1 cup mango or pineapple chunks

1. In a medium bowl, coat the chicken with the jerk marinade, cover, and refrigerate for 1 hour.

2. Spray a fryer basket lightly with olive oil.

3. Place the chicken in the fryer basket in a single layer and spray lightly with olive oil. You may need to cook the chicken in batches. Reserve any leftover marinade.

4. Air fry for 8 minutes. Turn the chicken over and brush with some of the remaining marinade. Cook until the chicken reaches an internal temperature of at least 165°F, an additional 5 to 7 minutes.

5. To assemble the wraps, fill each tortilla with ¼ cup carrots, ¼ cup cucumber, ¼ cup lettuce, and ¼ cup mango. Place one quarter of the chicken tenderloins on top and roll up the tortilla. These are great served warm or cold.

Make it Gluten-Free: Use gluten-free tortillas.

Per Serving

Calories: 325; Total Fat: 6g; Saturated Fat: 1g; Cholesterol: 65mg; Carbohydrates: 50g; Protein: 32g; Fiber: 15g; Sodium: 2,074mg

Spinach and Feta Chicken Meatballs

PREP TIME: 30 MINUTES / **COOK TIME:** 18 MINUTES / **SERVES** 6 / 350°F

Feta cheese adds a burst of flavor to these meatballs without adding a lot of extra calories, while spinach packs in a ton of vitamins, nutrients, and fiber, a key component in weight loss.

Olive oil
4 ounces fresh spinach, chopped
½ teaspoon salt, plus more as needed
½ cup whole-wheat panko bread crumbs
¼ teaspoon freshly ground black pepper
¼ teaspoon garlic powder
1 egg, beaten
1 pound lean ground chicken
⅓ cup crumbled feta cheese

1. Spray a large skillet lightly with olive oil. Add the spinach, season lightly with salt, and cook over medium heat until the spinach has wilted, 2 to 3 minutes. Set aside.

2. In a large bowl, mix together the panko bread crumbs, ½ teaspoon of salt, pepper, and garlic powder. Add the egg, chicken, spinach, and feta and stir to gently combine.

3. Using a heaping tablespoon, form 24 meatballs.

4. Lightly spray a fryer basket with olive oil.

5. Place the meatballs in the fryer basket in a single layer. Spray the meatballs lightly with olive oil. You may need to cook them in batches.

6. Air fry for 7 minutes. Turn the meatballs over and cook until golden brown, an additional 5 to 8 minutes.

Make It Dairy Free: You can mimic the salty flavor of feta cheese by replacing it with the same amount of finely diced kalamata olives.

Per Serving

Calories: 175; Total Fat: 9g; Saturated Fat: 3g; Cholesterol: 108mg; Carbohydrates: 6g; Protein: 19g; Fiber: 1g; Sodium: 409mg

Breaded Homestyle Chicken Strips

PREP TIME: 15 MINUTES / **COOK TIME:** 20 MINUTES / **SERVES** 4 / 370°F

Generations of people have fond memories of fried chicken strips, but they aren't the best food to eat when watching your waist. This air-fried rendition is healthier—whole-wheat bread crumbs are lower in net carbs than white flour coatings—and they still provide the crunch and flavor of the original. I call that a win!

DAIRY-FREE

1 tablespoon of olive oil, plus more for spraying
1 pound boneless, skinless chicken tenderloins
1 teaspoon salt
½ teaspoon freshly ground black pepper
½ teaspoon paprika
½ teaspoon garlic powder
½ cup whole-wheat seasoned bread crumbs
1 teaspoon dried parsley

1. Spray a fryer basket lightly with olive oil.

2. In a medium bowl, toss the chicken with the salt, pepper, paprika, and garlic powder until evenly coated.

3. Add the olive oil and toss to coat the chicken evenly.

4. In a separate, shallow bowl, mix together the bread crumbs and parsley.

5. Coat each piece of chicken evenly in the bread crumb mixture.

6. Place the chicken in the fryer basket in a single layer and spray it lightly with olive oil. You may need to cook them in batches.

7. Air fry for 10 minutes. Flip the chicken over, lightly spray with olive oil, and cook until golden brown, an additional 8 to 10 minutes.

Pair It With: For a kid-friendly meal serve with Broccoli Cheese Tots.

Per Serving

Calories: 178; Total Fat: 6g; Saturated Fat: 1g; Cholesterol: 65mg; Carbohydrates: 8g; Protein: 25g; Fiber: 1g; Sodium: 774mg

Black Pepper Chicken

PREP TIME: 10 MINUTES / **COOK TIME:** 15 MINUTES / **SERVES** 4 / 375°F

Hoisin sauce, a Chinese condiment, is the ingredient that gives this recipe its salty taste along with a little bit of sweetness, and adds a pop of flavor to a low-calorie meal. This recipe received the highest praise from my family and is on our regular meal rotation.

DAIRY-FREE

Olive oil
½ cup soy sauce
2 tablespoons hoisin sauce
4 teaspoons minced garlic
1 teaspoon freshly ground black pepper
8 boneless, skinless chicken tenderloins
1 cup chopped celery
1 medium red bell pepper, diced

1. Spray a fryer basket lightly with olive oil.

2. In a large bowl, mix together the soy sauce, hoisin sauce, garlic, and black pepper to make a marinade. Add the chicken, celery, and bell pepper and toss to coat.

3. Shake the excess marinade off the chicken, place it and the vegetables in the fryer basket, and lightly spray with olive oil. You may need to cook them in batches. Reserve the remaining marinade.

4. Air fry for 8 minutes. Turn the chicken over and brush with some of the remaining marinade. Cook until the chicken reaches an internal temperature of at least 165°F, an additional 5 to 7 minutes.

Pair It With: Serve with a side of Sweet and Spicy Broccoli.

Per Serving

Calories: 153; Total Fat: 1g; Saturated Fat: <1g; Cholesterol: 70mg; Carbohydrates: 10g; Protein: 27g; Fiber: 2g; Sodium: 2,123mg

Mexican Sheet Pan Dinner

PREP TIME: 10 MINUTES / **COOK TIME:** 15 MINUTES / **SERVES** 4 / 370°F

Traditionally cooked in the oven with all the vegetables and proteins combined on one sheet pan, this recipe takes those same ingredients and air fries them. Believe me, this will taste like chicken fajitas, but you won't need to clean up a messy frying pan. Serve with tortillas for a complete meal.

DAIRY-FREE

GLUTEN-FREE

1 pound boneless, skinless chicken tenderloins, cut into strips
3 bell peppers, any color, cut into chunks
1 onion, cut into chunks
1 tablespoon olive oil, plus more for spraying
1 tablespoon fajita seasoning mix

1. In a large bowl, mix together the chicken, bell peppers, onion, 1 tablespoon of olive oil, and fajita seasoning mix until completely coated.

2. Spray a fryer basket lightly with olive oil.

3. Place the chicken and vegetables in the fryer basket and lightly spray with olive oil.

4. Air fry for 7 minutes. Shake the basket and cook until the chicken is cooked through and the veggies are starting to char, an additional 5 to 8 minutes.

Air Fry Like a Pro: Make sure to cut the bell peppers and onions into the same size so they will cook evenly.

Per Serving

Calories: 178; Total Fat: 6g; Saturated Fat: 1g; Cholesterol: 65mg; Carbohydrates: 9g; Protein: 24g; Fiber: 2g; Sodium: 288mg

Parmesan-Lemon Chicken

PREP TIME: 1 HOUR 10 MINUTES / **COOK TIME:** 20 MINUTES / **SERVES** 4 / 360°F

Adding a small amount of Parmesan cheese to bread crumbs is a simple way to bring additional flavor to a protein. Parmesan cheese is also naturally low in fat, so it is a healthier choice than other cheeses.

1 egg
2 tablespoons lemon juice
2 teaspoons minced garlic
½ teaspoon salt
½ teaspoon freshly ground black pepper
4 boneless, skinless chicken breasts, thin cut
Olive oil
½ cup whole-wheat bread crumbs
¼ cup grated Parmesan cheese

1. In a medium bowl, whisk together the egg, lemon juice, garlic, salt, and pepper. Add the chicken breasts, cover, and refrigerate for up to 1 hour.

2. In a shallow bowl, combine the bread crumbs and Parmesan cheese.

3. Spray a fryer basket lightly with olive oil.

4. Remove the chicken breasts from the egg mixture, then dredge them in the bread crumb mixture, and place in the fryer basket in a single layer. Lightly spray the chicken breasts with olive oil. You may need to cook the chicken in batches.

5. Air fry for 8 minutes. Flip the chicken over, lightly spray with olive oil, and cook until the chicken reaches an internal temperature of 165°F, for an additional 7 to 12 minutes.

Air Fry Like a Pro: To get the best results when cooking chicken breasts, cut or pound them into thinner pieces, approximately ¾ inches thick. Otherwise the chicken could end up being overcooked on the outside while the inside is not completely cooked.

Per Serving

Calories: 195; Total Fat: 6g; Saturated Fat: 2g; Cholesterol: 116mg; Carbohydrates: 8g; Protein: 29g; Fiber: 1g; Sodium: 618mg

Italian Chicken and Veggies

PREP TIME: 10 MINUTES / **COOK TIME:** 30 MINUTES / **SERVES** 4 / 370°F TO 400°F

Balsamic vinaigrette dressing is an easy and delicious way to marinate chicken and vegetables without adding excessive calories or sodium. The green beans and grape tomatoes in this recipe add bright color (plus plenty of nourishing vitamins) to match.

GLUTEN-FREE

¾ cup balsamic vinaigrette dressing, divided
1 pound boneless, skinless chicken tenderloins
Olive oil
1 pound fresh green beans, trimmed
1 pint grape tomatoes

1. Place ½ cup of the balsamic vinaigrette dressing and the chicken in a large zip-top plastic bag, seal, and refrigerate for at least 1 hour or up to overnight.

2. In a large bowl, mix together the green beans, tomatoes, and the remaining ¼ cup of balsamic vinaigrette dressing until well coated.

3. Spray the fryer basket lightly with oil. Place the vegetables in the fryer basket. Reserve any remaining vinaigrette.

4. Air fry for 8 minutes. Shake the basket and continue to cook until the beans are crisp but tender, and the tomatoes are soft and slightly charred, an additional 5 to 7 minutes.

5. Wipe the fryer basket with a paper towel and spray lightly with olive oil.

6. Place the chicken in the fryer basket in a single layer. You may need to cook them in batches.

7. Air fry for 7 minutes. Flip the chicken over, baste with some of the remaining vinaigrette, and cook until the chicken reaches an internal temperature of 165°F, an additional 5 to 8 minutes.

8.   Serve the chicken and veggies together.

Per Serving

Calories: 266; Total Fat: 12g; Saturated Fat: 1g; Cholesterol: 65mg; Carbohydrates: 19g; Protein: 26g; Fiber: 5g; Sodium: 284mg

Whole Roasted Chicken

PREP TIME: 15 MINUTES / **COOK TIME:** 1 HOUR / **SERVES** 6 / 360°F

Your kitchen is going to smell divine when you make this. Roasting a whole chicken is so simple, and the end result is a healthy protein that's big enough to feed the whole family. Remember to shred any leftover meat and refrigerate or freeze it for future lunch bowls or wraps.

DAIRY-FREE

GLUTEN-FREE

Olive oil
1 teaspoon salt
1 teaspoon Italian seasoning
½ teaspoon freshly ground black pepper
½ teaspoon paprika
½ teaspoon garlic powder
½ teaspoon onion powder
2 tablespoons olive oil
1 (4-pound) fryer chicken

1. Spray a fryer basket lightly with olive oil.

2. In a small bowl, mix together the salt, Italian seasoning, pepper, paprika, garlic powder, and onion powder.

3. Remove any giblets from the chicken. Pat the chicken dry very thoroughly with paper towels, including the cavity.

4. Brush the chicken all over with the olive oil and rub it with the seasoning mixture.

5. Truss the chicken or tie the legs with butcher's twine. This will make it easier to flip the chicken during cooking.

6. Place the chicken in the fryer basket, breast side down. Air fry for 30 minutes. Flip the chicken over and baste it with any drippings collected in the bottom drawer of the air fryer. Lightly spray the chicken with olive oil.

7.   Air fry for 20 minutes. Flip the chicken over one last time and cook until a thermometer inserted into the thickest part of the thigh reaches at least 165°F and it's crispy and golden, 10 more minutes. Continue to cook, checking every 5 minutes until the chicken reaches the correct internal temperature.

8.   Let the chicken rest for 10 minutes before carving.

Per Serving

Calories: 435; Total Fat: 33g; Saturated Fat: 9g; Cholesterol: 140mg; Carbohydrates: 1g; Protein: 36g; Fiber: <1g; Sodium: 528mg

Creole Cornish Hens

PREP TIME: 10 MINUTES / **COOK TIME:** 40 MINUTES / **SERVES** 4 / 370°F

Cornish hens may sound overly fussy or fancy, but they are mouthwatering and a widely available protein that's extremely simple to cook. It's really just a smaller variety of chicken, and one Cornish hen makes a substantial single serving, or it can be shared between two people as a modest portion.

DAIRY-FREE

GLUTEN-FREE

2 tablespoons olive oil, plus more for spraying
½ tablespoon Creole seasoning
½ tablespoon garlic powder
½ tablespoon onion powder
½ tablespoon freshly ground black pepper
½ tablespoon paprika
2 Cornish hens

1. Spray a fryer basket lightly with olive oil.

2. In a small bowl, mix together the Creole seasoning, garlic powder, onion powder, pepper, and paprika.

3. Pat the Cornish hens dry and brush each hen all over with the 2 tablespoons of olive oil. Rub each hen with the seasoning mixture.

4. Place the Cornish hens in the fryer basket. Air fry for 15 minutes. Flip the hens over and baste with any drippings collected in the bottom drawer of the air fryer. Lightly spray them with olive oil.

5. Air fry for 15 minutes. Flip the hens back over and cook until a thermometer inserted into the thickest part of the thigh reaches at least 165°F and it's crispy and golden, an additional 5 to 10 minutes.

6. Let the hens rest for 10 minutes before carving.

Air Fry Like a Pro: Be sure to remove the basket holding the Cornish hens from the air fryer while they rest or they will continue to cook and end up tough.

Per Serving

Calories: 396; Total Fat: 30g; Saturated Fat: 8g; Cholesterol: 211mg; Carbohydrates: 2g; Protein: 31g; Fiber: 1g; Sodium: 572mg

Sweet and Spicy Turkey Meatballs

PREP TIME: 15 MINUTES / **COOK TIME:** 15 MINUTES / **SERVES** 6 / 350°F

Grab your basting brush and get ready to be wowed by the tantalizing taste of these glazed meatballs. In this recipe, you'll add the glaze halfway through the cooking time. These are so irresistible, your family won't even notice they're made from heart-healthy turkey.

DAIRY-FREE

Olive oil
1 pound lean ground turkey
½ cup whole-wheat panko bread crumbs
1 egg, beaten
1 tablespoon soy sauce
¼ cup plus 1 tablespoon hoisin sauce, divided
2 teaspoons minced garlic
⅛ teaspoon salt
⅛ teaspoon freshly ground black pepper
1 teaspoon sriracha

1. Spray a fryer basket lightly with olive oil.

2. In a large bowl, mix together the turkey, panko bread crumbs, egg, soy sauce, 1 tablespoon of hoisin sauce, garlic, salt, and black pepper.

3. Using a tablespoon, form 24 meatballs.

4. In a small bowl, combine the remaining ¼ cup of hoisin sauce and sriracha to make a glaze and set aside.

5. Place the meatballs in the fryer basket in a single layer. You may need to cook them in batches.

6. Air fry for 8 minutes. Brush the meatballs generously with the glaze and cook until cooked through, an additional 4 to 7 minutes.

Pair It With: Try them with a side of Roasted "Everything Bagel" Broccolini.

Per Serving

Calories: 175; Total Fat: 7g; Saturated Fat: 2g; Cholesterol: 85mg; Carbohydrates: 11g; Protein: 17g; Fiber: 1g; Sodium: 485mg

Stuffed Bell Peppers

PREP TIME: 20 MINUTES / **COOK TIME:** 15 MINUTES / **SERVES** 4 / 360°F

These easy stuffed peppers have a Mexican-inspired flair. Packed with extra protein from the ground turkey and black beans, these are sure to fill you up fast without overloading you with calories. Long grain brown rice is one of the healthiest rice choices because it's lower on the glycemic index and contains more fiber than white rice.

GLUTEN-FREE

½ pound lean ground turkey
4 medium bell peppers
1 (15-ounce) can black beans, drained and rinsed
1 cup shredded reduced-fat Cheddar cheese
1 cup cooked long-grain brown rice
1 cup mild salsa
1¼ teaspoons chili powder
1 teaspoon salt
½ teaspoon ground cumin
½ teaspoon freshly ground black pepper
Olive oil
Chopped fresh cilantro, for garnish

1. In a large skillet over medium-high heat, cook the turkey, breaking it up with a spoon, until browned, about 5 minutes. Drain off any excess fat.

2. Cut about ½ inch off the tops of the peppers and then cut in half lengthwise. Remove and discard the seeds and set the peppers aside.

3. In a large bowl, combine the browned turkey, black beans, Cheddar cheese, rice, salsa, chili powder, salt, cumin, and black pepper. Spoon the mixture into the bell peppers.

4. Lightly spray a fryer basket with olive oil.

5. Place the stuffed peppers in the fryer basket. Air fry until heated throughout, 10 to 15 minutes. Garnish with cilantro and serve.

Make It Even Lower Calorie: If you are watching your carbohydrate intake closely and want to lower calories and carbs, replace the rice with a cup of halved cherry tomatoes.

Per Serving

Calories: 391; Total Fat: 12g; Saturated Fat: 5g; Cholesterol: 60mg; Carbohydrates: 48g; Protein: 28g; Fiber: 11g; Sodium: 1,206mg

Hoisin Turkey Burgers

PREP TIME: 40 MINUTES / **COOK TIME:** 20 MINUTES / **SERVES** 4 / 370°F

Turkey burgers have an unfair reputation for being boring, but it only takes a few extra ingredients to add zing to your patty. These are lower in calories and fat than their ground beef counterparts and they offer bold flavor.

DAIRY-FREE

Olive oil
1 pound lean ground turkey
¼ cup whole-wheat bread crumbs
¼ cup hoisin sauce
2 tablespoons soy sauce
4 whole-wheat buns

1. Spray a fryer basket lightly with olive oil.

2. In a large bowl, mix together the turkey, bread crumbs, hoisin sauce, and soy sauce.

3. Form the mixture into 4 equal patties. Cover with plastic wrap and refrigerate the patties for 30 minutes.

4. Place the patties in the fryer basket in a single layer. Spray the patties lightly with olive oil.

5. Air fry for 10 minutes. Flip the patties over, lightly spray with olive oil, and cook until golden brown, an additional 5 to 10 minutes.

6. Place the patties on buns and top with your choice of low-calorie burger toppings like sliced tomatoes, onions, and cabbage slaw.

Per Serving

Calories: 347; Total Fat: 11g; Saturated Fat: 3g; Cholesterol: 81mg; Carbohydrates: 35g; Protein: 30g; Fiber: 5g; Sodium: 990mg

Easy Turkey Tenderloin

PREP TIME: 20 MINUTES / **COOK TIME:** 30 MINUTES / **SERVES** 4 / 370°F

This recipe couldn't be easier for when you're short on prep time. If you have a turkey breast tenderloin and some very basic spices on hand, you're good to go. The air fryer keeps the meat tender and juicy without adding fat, while the minimal spicing really helps its subtle flavor shine.

DAIRY-FREE

GLUTEN-FREE

Olive oil
½ teaspoon paprika
½ teaspoon garlic powder
½ teaspoon salt
½ teaspoon freshly ground black pepper
Pinch cayenne pepper
1½ pound turkey breast tenderloin

1. Spray a fryer basket lightly with olive oil.

2. In a small bowl, combine the paprika, garlic powder, salt, black pepper, and cayenne pepper. Rub the mixture all over the turkey.

3. Place the turkey in the fryer basket and lightly spray with olive oil.

4. Air fry for 15 minutes. Flip the turkey over and lightly spray with olive oil. Air fry until the internal temperature reaches at least 170°F for an additional 10 to 15 minutes.

5. Let the turkey rest for 10 minutes before slicing and serving.

Pair It With: Keep dinner simple by serving with Green Beans and New Potatoes.

Per Serving

Calories: 183; Total Fat: 1g; Saturated Fat: 0g; Cholesterol: 105mg; Carbohydrates: 1g; Protein: 42g; Fiber: <1g; Sodium: 374mg

Apricot-Glazed Turkey Tenderloin

PREP TIME: 20 MINUTES / **COOK TIME:** 30 MINUTES / **SERVES** 4 / 370°F

Sugar-free preserves are my secret weapon for creating a sweet and savory glaze without the extra sugar. If you can't find apricot preserves, try substituting orange marmalade or even apple jelly in this recipe. These ingredients combine delightfully with the spicy brown mustard for just the right combination of sweet and savory.

DAIRY-FREE

GLUTEN-FREE

Olive oil
¼ cup sugar-free apricot preserves
½ tablespoon spicy brown mustard
1½ pound turkey breast tenderloin
Salt
Freshly ground black pepper

1. Spray a fryer basket lightly with olive oil.

2. In a small bowl, combine the apricot preserves and mustard to make a paste.

3. Season the turkey with salt and pepper. Spread the apricot paste all over the turkey.

4. Place the turkey in the fryer basket and lightly spray with olive oil.

5. Air fry for 15 minutes. Flip the turkey over and lightly spray with olive oil. Air fry until the internal temperature reaches at least 170°F, an additional 10 to 15 minutes.

6. Let the turkey rest for 10 minutes before slicing and serving.

Pair It With: For a satisfying meal, make a side of Crunchy Hasselback Potatoes.

Per Serving

Calories: 192; Total Fat: 1g; Saturated Fat: 0g; Cholesterol: 105mg; Carbohydrates: 5g; Protein: 42g; Fiber: 0g; Sodium: 113mg

Herb-Roasted Turkey Breast

PREP TIME: 20 MINUTES / **COOK TIME:** 45 MINUTES / **SERVES** 6 / 370°F

I love to stock my refrigerator with high-quality, low-fat proteins, so that I'll reach for them first come dinnertime. Turkey breast has less fat and calories than most other cuts of meat, and it absorbs spices easily. The herb rub in this recipe will fill your kitchen with the comforting scents of the Mediterranean.

GLUTEN-FREE

1 tablespoon olive oil, plus more for spraying
2 garlic cloves, minced
2 teaspoons Dijon mustard
1½ teaspoons rosemary
1½ teaspoons sage
1½ teaspoons thyme
1 teaspoon salt
½ teaspoon freshly ground black pepper
3 pounds turkey breast, thawed if frozen

1. Spray a fryer basket lightly with olive oil.

2. In a small bowl, mix together the garlic, olive oil, Dijon mustard, rosemary, sage, thyme, salt, and pepper to make a paste. Smear the paste all over the turkey breast.

3. Place the turkey breast in the fryer basket.

4. Air fry for 20 minutes. Flip turkey breast over and baste it with any drippings that have collected in the bottom drawer of the air fryer. Air fry until the internal temperature of the meat reaches at least 170°F, 20 more minutes.

5. If desired, increase the temperature to 400°F, flip the turkey breast over one last time, and air fry for up to 5 minutes to get a crispy exterior.

6. Let the turkey rest for 10 minutes before slicing and serving.

Per Serving

Calories: 267; Total Fat: 3g; Saturated Fat: <1g; Cholesterol: 140mg; Carbohydrates: 1g; Protein: 56g; Fiber: 1g; Sodium: 538mg

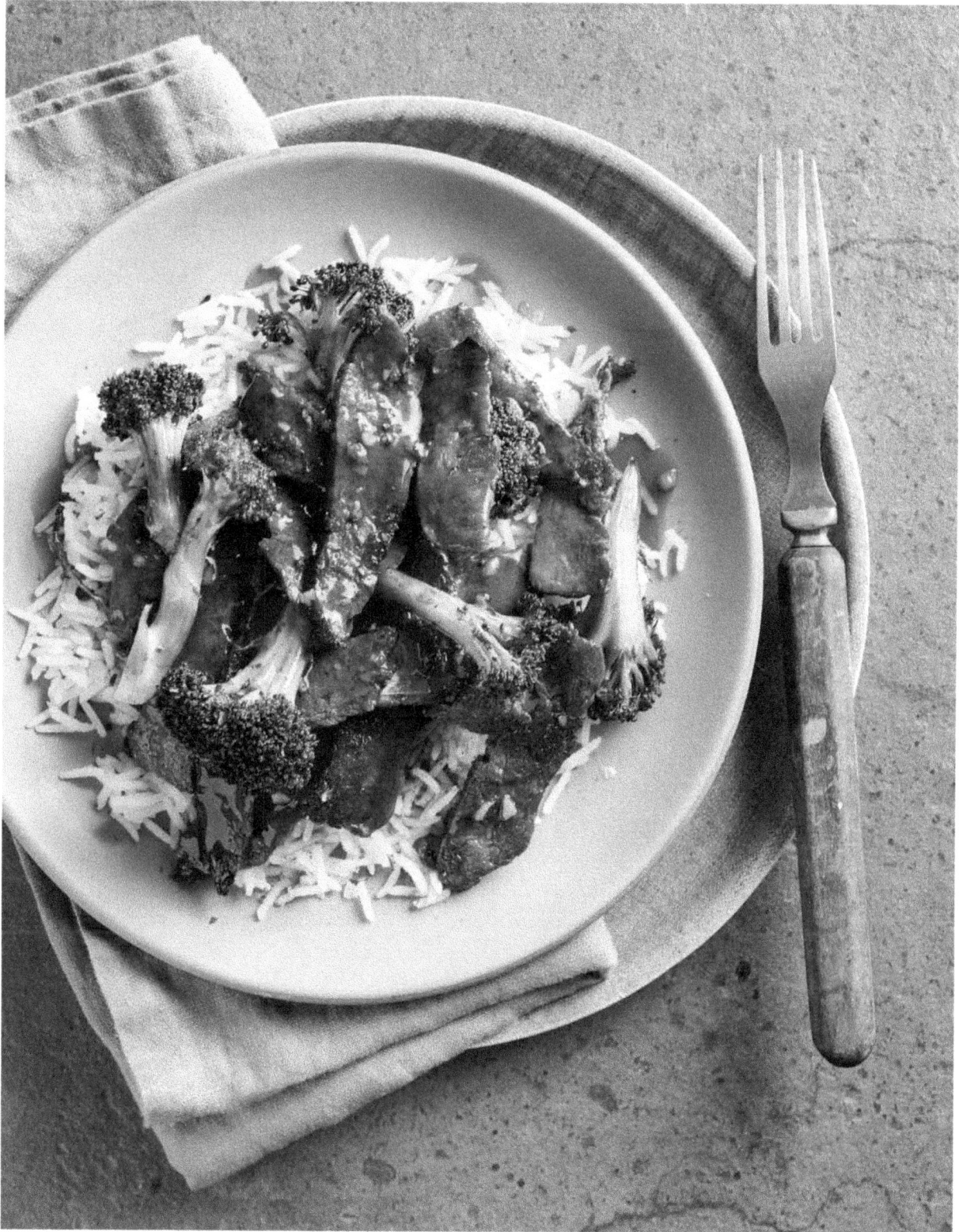
BEEF AND BROCCOLI STIR FRY

CHAPTER 8

Beef and Pork

Blue Cheese Burgers

Cheeseburger-Stuffed Bell Peppers

Mini Meatloaves

Beef and Mushroom Meatballs

Steak and Veggie Kebabs

Steak and Mushroom Bites

Beef and Broccoli Stir Fry

Korean BBQ Beef Bowls

Beef and Bean Chimichangas

Steak Fingers

Beef Roll-Ups

Rib Eye Steak

Pork and Apple Skewers

Mesquite Pork Medallions

Breaded Pork Cutlets

Chili-Lime Pork Loin

Sweet and Spicy Pork Chops

Breaded Italian Pork Chops

Pork and Ginger Meatball Bowl

Hawaiian Pork Sliders

Blue Cheese Burgers

PREP TIME: 10 MINUTES / **COOK TIME:** 20 MINUTES / **SERVES** 4 / 360°F

Just a little bit of blue cheese adds a lot of tang to these burgers, and eating smaller amounts of cheese is always a good thing when it comes to weight loss. Hot sauce, garlic, and Worcestershire add extra layers of flavor, meaning you won't have to drown your patty in sugary ketchup.

Olive oil
1 pound lean ground beef
½ cup blue cheese, crumbled
1 teaspoon Worcestershire sauce
½ teaspoon freshly ground black pepper
½ teaspoon hot sauce
½ teaspoon minced garlic
¼ teaspoon salt
4 whole-wheat buns

1. Spray a fryer basket lightly with olive oil.

2. In a large bowl, mix together the beef, blue cheese, Worcestershire sauce, pepper, hot sauce, garlic, and salt.

3. Form the mixture into 4 patties.

4. Place the patties in the fryer basket in a single layer, leaving a little room between them for even cooking.

5. Air fry for 10 minutes. Flip over and cook until the meat reaches an internal temperature of at least 160°F, an additional 7 to 10 minutes.

6. Place each patty on a bun and serve with low-calorie toppings like sliced tomatoes or onions.

Pair It With: Avocado Fries go great with these burgers.

Per Serving

Calories: 373; Total Fat: 14g; Saturated Fat: 7g; Cholesterol: 78mg; Carbohydrates: 25g; Protein: 34g; Fiber: 4g; Sodium: 657mg

Cheeseburger-Stuffed Bell Peppers

PREP TIME: 15 MINUTES / **COOK TIME:** 20 MINUTES / **SERVES** 4 / 360°F

Stuffed bell peppers make a great all-in-one dinner. This cheeseburger version is my favorite filling, but you can combine whatever flavors you like best. The best part? No bun means fewer calories.

GLUTEN-FREE

Olive oil
4 large red bell peppers
1 pound lean ground beef
1 cup diced onion
Salt
Freshly ground black pepper
1 cup cooked brown rice
½ cup shredded reduced-fat Cheddar cheese
½ cup tomato sauce
2 tablespoons dill pickle relish
2 tablespoons ketchup
1 tablespoon Worcestershire sauce
1 tablespoon mustard
½ cup shredded lettuce
½ cup diced tomatoes

1. Spray a fryer basket lightly with olive oil.

2. Cut about ½ inch off the tops of the peppers. Remove any seeds from the insides. Set aside.

3. In a large skillet over medium-high heat, cook the ground beef and onion until browned, about 5 minutes. Season with salt and pepper.

4. In a large bowl, mix together the ground beef mixture, rice, Cheddar cheese, tomato sauce, relish, ketchup, Worcestershire sauce, and mustard.

5. Spoon the meat and rice mixture equally into the peppers.

6. Place the stuffed peppers into the fryer basket. Air fry until golden brown

on top, 10 to 15 minutes.

7.   Top each pepper with the shredded lettuce and diced tomatoes and serve.

Make it Dairy Free: Either leave the cheese out completely or use a shredded dairy-free cheese.

Per Serving

Calories: 366; Total Fat: 11g; Saturated Fat: 5g; Cholesterol: 75mg; Carbohydrates: 33g; Protein: 32g; Fiber: 6g; Sodium: 612mg

Mini Meatloaves

PREP TIME: 10 MINUTES / **COOK TIME:** 20 MINUTES / **SERVES** 4 / 350°F

Few dishes are more comforting than meatloaf. It originated as a result of thrifty home cooks trying to stretch food budgets further by adding fillers to meat. Meatloaf can be high in calories, but here I've made it weight loss–friendly by using lean ground beef and low-fat milk, while the mini loaf size will help with portion control.

Olive oil
1 pound lean ground beef
1 egg, beaten
1 cup whole-wheat bread crumbs
¼ cup low-fat evaporated milk
¼ cup plus 2 tablespoons barbeque sauce, divided
1 teaspoon onion powder
1 teaspoon salt
½ teaspoon freshly ground black pepper

1. Spray a fryer basket lightly with olive oil.

2. In a large bowl, mix together the ground beef, egg, bread crumbs, milk, ¼ cup of barbeque sauce, onion powder, salt, and pepper and mix well.

3. Divide the beef mixture into four small meatloaf shapes. Spread ½ tablespoon of the remaining barbeque sauce on top of each mini meatloaf.

4. Place the meatloaves in the fryer basket in a single layer. Air fry until the internal temperature reaches at least 160°F, 15 to 20 minutes.

Make it Gluten-Free: You can substitute 1 cup of gluten-free quick oats in place of the bread crumbs.

Per Serving

Calories: 306; Total Fat: 9g; Saturated Fat: 4g; Cholesterol: 112mg; Carbohydrates: 19g; Protein: 30g; Fiber: 3g; Sodium: 902mg

Beef and Mushroom Meatballs

PREP TIME: 15 MINUTES / **COOK TIME:** 15 MINUTES / **SERVES** 6 / 390°F

Meatballs are a family favorite, and when you add the earthy flavor of mushrooms, they become a lower-calorie comfort food you'll love on a chilly night. They are also an ideal party food—simply pop a toothpick in each one and serve them on a platter.

DAIRY-FREE

Olive oil
2 pounds lean ground beef
⅔ cups finely chopped mushrooms
4 tablespoons chopped parsley
2 eggs, beaten
2 teaspoons salt
1 teaspoon freshly ground black pepper
1 cup whole-wheat bread crumbs

1. Spray a fryer basket lightly with olive oil.

2. In a large bowl, mix together the beef, mushrooms, and parsley. Add the eggs, salt, and pepper and mix gently. Add the bread crumbs and mix until the bread crumbs are no longer dry. Be careful not to overmix.

3. Using a small cookie scoop, form 24 meatballs.

4. Place the meatballs in the fryer basket in a single layer and spray lightly with olive oil. You may need to cook the meatballs in batches.

5. Air fry until the internal temperature reaches at least 160°F, 10 to 15 minutes, shaking the basket every 5 minutes for even cooking.

Pair It With: Crunchy Hasselback Potatoes are the perfect accompaniment and will complete a hearty, satisfying meal.

Per Serving

Calories: 314; Total Fat: 11g; Saturated Fat: 5g; Cholesterol: 149mg; Carbohydrates: 10g; Protein: 37g; Fiber: 2g; Sodium: 909mg

Steak and Veggie Kebabs

PREP TIME: 10 MINUTES, PLUS 2 HOURS TO MARINATE / **COOK TIME:** 15 MINUTES / **SERVES** 4 / 350°F

Kebabs are a convenient way to cook meat and vegetables together at the same time. You will need skewers that fit into the air fryer, and if they are wooden, soak them in water for at least 30 minutes before using.

DAIRY-FREE

½ cup soy sauce
3 tablespoons lemon juice
2 tablespoons Worcestershire sauce
2 tablespoons Dijon mustard
1 teaspoon minced garlic
¾ teaspoon freshly ground black pepper
1 pound sirloin steak, cut into 1-inch cubes
1 medium red bell pepper, cut into big chunks
1 medium green bell pepper, cut into big chunks
1 medium red onion, cut into big chunks
Olive oil

1. In a small bowl, whisk together the soy sauce, lemon juice, Worcestershire sauce, Dijon mustard, garlic, and black pepper. Divide the marinade equally between two large zip-top plastic bags.

2. Place the steak in one of the bags, seal, and refrigerate for at least 2 hours. Place the vegetables in the other bag, seal, and refrigerate for 1 hour.

3. If using wooden skewers, soak the skewers in water for at least 30 minutes.

4. Spray a fryer basket lightly with olive oil.

5. Thread the steak and veggies alternately onto the skewers.

6. Place the skewers in the fryer basket in a single layer. You may need to cook the skewers in batches.

7. Air fry for 8 minutes. Flip the skewers over, lightly spray with olive oil, and cook until the steak reaches your desired level of doneness, an additional 4

to 7 minutes. The internal temperature should read 125°F for rare, 135°F for medium rare, 145°F for medium and 150°F for medium well.

Per Serving

Calories: 271; Total Fat: 7g; Saturated Fat: 3g; Cholesterol: 65mg; Carbohydrates: 12g; Protein: 38g; Fiber: 2g; Sodium: 2,147mg

Steak and Mushroom Bites

PREP TIME: 5 MINUTES, PLUS 1 HOUR TO MARINATE / **COOK TIME:** 20 MINUTES /
SERVES 4 / 400°F

I have always loved the combination of steak and mushrooms. To get the full
health benefits of mushrooms they should be cooked, because mushrooms have
tough cell walls that make it difficult for the digestive system to break them
down and gain access to all the nutrients. Cooking softens the walls and the
body can digest them more easily.

DAIRY-FREE

1 pound sirloin steak, cut into ½ inch cubes
8 ounces mushrooms, sliced
1 tablespoon Worcestershire sauce
1 tablespoon balsamic vinegar
1 tablespoon soy sauce
1 tablespoon olive oil, plus more for spraying
1 teaspoon Dijon mustard
1 teaspoon minced garlic
Salt
Freshly ground black pepper

1. Place the steak and mushrooms in a large zip-top plastic bag. Add the
   Worcestershire sauce, balsamic vinegar, soy sauce, olive oil, Dijon mustard,
   and garlic. Season to taste with salt and pepper, seal, and refrigerate for at
   least 1 hour or overnight.

2. Spray a fryer basket lightly with olive oil.

3. Add the steak and mushrooms to the fryer basket in an even layer. You may
   need to cook in batches.

4. Air fry for 10 minutes. Shake the basket and cook until the steak reaches
   your desired level of doneness, an additional 5 to 10 minutes. The internal
   temperature should read 125°F for rare, 135°F for medium rare, 145°F for
   medium and 150°F for medium well.

Make it Gluten-Free: Replace the soy sauce with 1 additional tablespoon of

Worcestershire sauce.

Calories: 261; Total Fat: 10g; Saturated Fat: 3g; Cholesterol: 65mg; Carbohydrates: 4g; Protein: 37g; Fiber: 1g; Sodium: 378mg

Beef and Broccoli Stir Fry

PREP TIME: 15 MINUTES, PLUS 2 HOURS TO MARINATE / **COOK TIME:** 15 MINUTES / **SERVES** 4 / 370°F

Restaurant-style beef and broccoli tends to be high in fat, sodium, and hidden sugars. Learning to make this beloved dish with its lean protein and plenty of fresh broccoli at home is a much healthier option.

DAIRY-FREE

3 tablespoons dry sherry
¼ cup soy sauce
4 garlic cloves, minced
1 tablespoon sesame oil
½ teaspoon red pepper flakes
1 pound flank or skirt steak, trimmed and cut into strips
Olive oil
½ pound broccoli florets
¼ cup beef broth
2 teaspoons cornstarch

1. In a small bowl, combine the sherry, soy sauce, garlic, sesame oil, and red pepper flakes to create a marinade.

2. Place the steak and 3 tablespoons of the marinade in a large zip-top plastic bag, seal, and refrigerate for at least 2 hours.

3. Spray a fryer basket lightly with olive oil.

4. Add half the steak to the fryer basket along with half the broccoli florets. Lightly spray with olive oil.

5. Air fry for 8 minutes. Shake the basket to redistribute and cook until cooked through, an additional 4 to 7 minutes. Repeat with the remaining steak and broccoli. Transfer the steak and broccoli to a large bowl.

6. While the steak is cooking, in a small saucepan over medium-high heat, combine the broth and remaining marinade and bring to a boil.

7. In a small bowl combine the cornstarch and 1 tablespoon of water to create

a slurry. Add the slurry to the sauce pan and simmer, stirring, until the sauce starts to thicken, a few seconds to 1 minute.

8. Pour the sauce over the cooked steak and broccoli and toss to evenly coat.

Serve It With: Spoon the stir fry over steamed rice for a heartier meal.

Per Serving

Calories: 259; Total Fat: 11g; Saturated Fat: 1g; Cholesterol: 45mg; Carbohydrates: 9g; Protein: 27g; Fiber: 2g; Sodium: 1,016mg

Korean BBQ Beef Bowls

PREP TIME: 10 MINUTES, PLUS UP TO 2 HOURS TO MARINATE / **COOK TIME:** 25 MINUTES / **SERVES** 4 / 380°F

Vinegar has a high acid content that can really brighten the flavor of foods when they are cooking. Although there is no sodium in vinegar, it can serve as a substitute for salt in many recipes. Sesame oil is high in antioxidants and has anti-inflammatory properties.

DAIRY-FREE

½ cup soy sauce
2 tablespoons brown sugar
2 tablespoons red wine vinegar or rice vinegar
1 tablespoon olive oil, plus more for spraying
1 tablespoon sesame oil
1 pound flank steak, sliced very thin against the grain
2 teaspoons cornstarch
2 cups cooked brown rice
2 cups steamed broccoli florets

1. In a large bowl, whisk together the soy sauce, brown sugar, vinegar, olive oil, and sesame oil. Add the steak, cover with plastic wrap, and refrigerate for at least 30 minutes or up to 2 hours.

2. Spray a fryer basket lightly with olive oil.

3. Remove as much marinade as possible from the steak. Reserve any leftover marinade.

4. Place the steak in the fryer basket in a single layer. You may need to cook the steak in batches.

5. Air fry for 10 minutes. Flip the steak over and cook until the steak reaches your desired level of doneness, an additional 7 to 10 minutes. The internal temperature should read 125°F for rare, 135°F for medium rare, 145°F for medium, and 150°F for medium well. Transfer the steak to a large bowl and set aside.

6. While the steak is cooking, in a small saucepan over medium-high heat, bring the remaining marinade to a boil.

7. In a small bowl, combine the cornstarch and 1 tablespoon of water to create a slurry. Add the slurry to the marinade, lower the heat to medium-low, and simmer, stirring, until the sauce starts to thicken, a few seconds to 1 minute.

8. Pour the sauce over the steak and stir to combine.

9. To assemble the bowls, spoon ½ cup brown rice and ½ cup of broccoli into each of four bowls and top with the steak.

Air Fry Like a Pro: If you cut your own flank steak you can control how thin you'd like the slices. When you buy pre-cut stir fry beef strips from the butcher, they will likely be thicker than I recommend and may require a few additional minutes of cooking time. Keep an eye on the cooking time and check to make sure the meat reaches at least 145°F.

Per Serving

Calories: 399; Total Fat: 15g; Saturated Fat: 1g; Cholesterol: 45mg; Carbohydrates: 36g; Protein: 29g; Fiber: 3g; Sodium: 1,875mg

Beef and Bean Chimichangas

PREP TIME: 15 MINUTES / **COOK TIME:** 15 MINUTES / **SERVES** 4 / 360°F

A restaurant-style fried chimichanga can top out at well over 20 grams of fat. Making your own chimichangas at home in the air fryer will cut that down. It also allows you to choose fat-free beans and low-fat cheese options.

Olive oil
1 pound lean ground beef
1 tablespoon taco seasoning
½ cup salsa
1 (16-ounce) can fat-free refried beans
4 large whole-wheat tortillas
½ cup shredded Cheddar cheese

1. Spray fryer basket lightly with olive oil.

2. In a large skillet over medium heat, cook the ground beef until browned, about 5 minutes. Add the taco seasoning and salsa and stir to combine. Set aside.

3. Spread ½ cup of refried beans onto each tortilla, leaving a ½ inch border around the edge. Add ¼ of the ground beef mixture to each tortilla and sprinkle with 2 tablespoons of Cheddar cheese.

4. Fold the opposite sides of the tortilla in and roll up.

5. Place the chimichangas in the fryer basket, seam side down. Spray lightly with olive oil. You may need to cook the chimichangas in batches.

6. Air fry until golden brown, 5 to 10 minutes.

Make it Gluten-Free: Delicious gluten-free tortillas are available in most grocery stores these days.

Per Serving

Calories: 532; Total Fat: 16g; Saturated Fat: 7g; Cholesterol: 78mg; Carbohydrates: 50g; Protein: 40g; Fiber: 12g; Sodium: 1,292mg

Steak Fingers

PREP TIME: 15 MINUTES / **COOK TIME:** 15 MINUTES / **SERVES** 4 / 360°F

Cube steaks are a cut of beef that has been tenderized and flattened prior to purchase and are made with leaner cuts of beef such as top round or top sirloin. They have little to no fat marbling, so they make a great choice when trying to lose weight.

Olive oil
½ cup whole-wheat flour
1 teaspoon seasoned salt
½ teaspoon freshly ground black pepper
¼ teaspoon cayenne pepper
2 eggs, beaten
½ cup low-fat milk
1 pound cube steaks, cut into 1-inch-wide strips

1. Spray a fryer basket lightly with olive oil.

2. In a shallow bowl, mix together the flour, salt, black pepper, and cayenne.

3. In another shallow bowl, whisk together the eggs and milk.

4. Dredge the steak strips in the flour mixture, coat with the egg mixture, and dredge in the flour mixture once more to coat completely.

5. Place the steak strips in the fryer basket in a single layer and spray lightly with olive oil. You may need to cook the steak in batches.

6. Air fry for 8 minutes. Flip the steak strips over and lightly spray with olive oil. Cook until golden brown and crispy, an additional 4 to 7 minutes.

Per Serving

Calories: 288; Total Fat: 12g; Saturated Fat: 5g; Cholesterol: 175mg; Carbohydrates: 13g; Protein: 30g; Fiber: 2g; Sodium: 700mg

Beef Roll-Ups

PREP TIME: 30 MINUTES, PLUS 30 MINUTES TO MARINATE / **COOK TIME:** 20 MINUTES / **SERVES** 4 / 400°F

Sirloin steaks tend to be lean, juicy, and tender, and they are also one of the more affordable cuts of beef. Using a meat mallet to flatten them makes them even more tender. Many beef roll-up recipes require cooking the peppers separately. Making these in the air fryer removes that step, producing slightly crunchy peppers inside a perfectly cooked steak. You will need wooden toothpicks to hold the rolls together.

GLUTEN-FREE

1½ pounds sirloin steak, cut into slices
2 tablespoons Worcestershire sauce
½ tablespoon garlic powder
½ tablespoon onion powder
2 medium bell peppers of any color, cut into thin strips
½ cup shredded mozzarella cheese
Salt
Freshly ground black pepper
Olive oil

1. Using a meat mallet, pound the steaks very thin.

2. In a small bowl, combine the Worcestershire sauce, garlic powder, and onion powder to make a marinade.

3. Place the steaks and marinade in a large zip-top plastic bag, seal, and refrigerate for at least 30 minutes.

4. Soak 8 toothpicks in water for 15 to 20 minutes.

5. Place ¼ of the bell peppers and ¼ of the mozzarella cheese in the center of each steak. Season with salt and black pepper. Roll each steak up tightly and secure with 2 toothpicks.

6. Spray a fryer basket lightly with olive oil. Place the beef roll-ups in the fryer basket, toothpick side down, in a single layer. You may need to cook the

roll-ups in batches.

7. Air fry for 10 minutes. Flip the steaks over and cook until the meat reaches an internal temperature of at least 150°F, an additional 7 to 10 minutes.

8. Let the roll-ups rest for 10 minutes before serving.

Per Serving

Calories: 378; Total Fat: 13g; Saturated Fat: 6g; Cholesterol: 106mg; Carbohydrates: 7g; Protein: 56g; Fiber: 1g; Sodium: 297mg

Rib Eye Steak

PREP TIME: 5 MINUTES / **COOK TIME:** 15 MINUTES / **SERVES** 4 / 400°F

When you make steak in the air fryer, you don't have to worry about prepping a grill or smoking up your house by cooking them in a cast-iron pan. These rib eyes come out perfect with simple seasonings and a little olive oil—there's no marinating necessary—and steak will be cooked consistently every time.

DAIRY-FREE

GLUTEN-FREE

Olive oil
2 (8 ounce) rib eye steaks
1 tablespoon olive oil
1 teaspoon garlic salt
Salt
Freshly ground black pepper

1. Spray a fryer basket lightly with olive oil.

2. Drizzle olive oil over both sides of the steaks. Season both sides of the steaks with the garlic salt, salt, and pepper and massage the seasonings into the meat.

3. Place the steaks in the fryer basket in a single layer. You may need to cook the steaks in two batches.

4. Air fry at for 6 minutes. Flip the steaks over and cook until steak reaches your desired level of doneness, an additional 5 to 9 minutes. The steak should be at least 125°F for rare, 135°F for medium rare, 145°F for medium, and 150°F for medium well.

Pair It With: Spiced Balsamic Asparagus makes a steakhouse-worthy side to these rib eyes.

Per Serving

Calories: 207; Total Fat: 13g; Saturated Fat: 4g; Cholesterol: 67mg; Carbohydrates: 0g; Protein: 23g; Fiber: 0g; Sodium: 422mg

Pork and Apple Skewers

PREP TIME: 15 MINUTES / **COOK TIME:** 20 MINUTES / **SERVES** 4 / 350°F TO 370°F

Pork and apples complement each other perfectly. Here, the natural sweetness of the apples combined with the zesty glaze will have you asking for a second helping. You will need skewers that fit into the air fryer and if they are wooden, soak them in water for at least 30 minutes before using.

DAIRY-FREE

GLUTEN-FREE

For the glaze
½ cup sugar-free apricot preserves
3 tablespoons lemon juice
2 tablespoons Dijon mustard
2 teaspoons dried rosemary
1 teaspoon lemon zest

For the kebabs
Olive oil
2 gala apples, cored and sliced into wedges
1 pound pork tenderloin, cut into 1-inch pieces
Salt
Freshly ground black pepper

To make the glaze

1. In a small bowl, whisk together the apricot preserves, lemon juice, Dijon mustard, rosemary, and lemon zest. Set aside.

To make the kebabs

2. Spray a fryer basket lightly with olive oil.

3. Cut each wedge of apple in half crosswise into chunks.

4. If using wooden skewers, soak them in water for at least 30 minutes before using.

5. Thread the pork and apples alternately onto the skewers. Spray lightly all

over with olive oil and season with salt and pepper.

6. Place the skewers in the fryer basket in a single layer. You may need to cook the skewers in batches.

7. Air fry for 10 minutes. Generously brush the glaze onto the skewers.

8. Increase the temperature to 370°F and air fry for 5 minutes. Flip the skewers over, baste again with the glaze, and cook until the pork reaches an internal temperature of at least 145°F, an additional 3 to 5 minutes.

Per Serving

Calories: 200; Total Fat: 3g; Saturated Fat: 1g; Cholesterol: 45mg; Carbohydrates: 25g; Protein: 24g; Fiber: 3g; Sodium: 254mg

Mesquite Pork Medallions

PREP TIME: 10 MINUTES / **COOK TIME:** 20 MINUTES / **SERVES** 5 / 360°F

A lean protein that's low in fat and provides B vitamins, pork tenderloin cooks quickly, making it a welcome dinner option on busy weeknights. The mesquite seasoning gives it a classic BBQ-inspired flavor. Because pork is so mild tasting, it's an ideal vehicle for experimentation—try using za'atar, Italian seasoning, or a mustard-forward spice rub.

DAIRY-FREE

GLUTEN-FREE

2 teaspoons olive oil, plus more for spraying
1 pound boneless pork tenderloin
2 tablespoons mesquite seasoning

1. Spray a fryer basket lightly with olive oil.

2. Pat the pork dry with a paper towel. Cut it into 10 (½-inch) medallions.

3. In a medium bowl, toss the pork with the mesquite seasoning and coat with the olive oil.

4. Place the pork in the fryer basket in a single layer, leaving room between each medallion. You may need to cook them in batches.

5. Air fry for 10 minutes. Flip the pork over and lightly spray with olive oil. Cook until the pork reaches an internal temperature of at least 145°F, an additional 7 to 10 minutes.

Per Serving

Calories: 124; Total Fat: 4g; Saturated Fat: 1g; Cholesterol: 36mg; Carbohydrates: 3g; Protein: 19g; Fiber: 0g; Sodium: 206mg

Breaded Pork Cutlets

PREP TIME: 15 MINUTES / **COOK TIME:** 15 MINUTES / **SERVES** 4 / 400°F

Breaded pork cutlets are traditionally fried in hot oil, making it a high-calorie treat. In this recipe, cooking them in the air fryer gives them an equally crispy exterior (and tender interior) without all those unwanted saturated fats.

DAIRY-FREE

Olive oil
½ cup whole wheat-panko bread crumbs
½ teaspoon garlic powder
2 eggs, beaten
4 (1-inch) boneless pork chops, fat trimmed
Salt
Freshly ground black pepper

1. Spray a fryer basket lightly with olive oil.

2. In a shallow bowl, mix together the panko bread crumbs and garlic powder.

3. In another shallow bowl, whisk the eggs with 1 teaspoon of water.

4. Place the pork chops between two sheets of parchment paper or plastic wrap. Using a meat mallet or a rolling pin, pound the pork chops until they are ¼ inch thick. Season them with salt and pepper.

5. Coat the pork in the egg mixture and shake off any excess, then dredge them in the bread crumb mixture.

6. Place the pork in the fryer basket in a single layer. Lightly spray the pork cutlets with olive oil. You may need to cook them in batches.

7. Air fry for 8 minutes. Flip the pork cutlets and lightly spray with olive oil. Cook until the pork reaches an internal temperature of at least 145°F, an additional 4 to 7 minutes.

Air Fry Like a Pro: It is important to try to pound the pork chops into equally thick cutlets for even cooking in the air fryer.

Per Serving

Calories: 212; Total Fat: 8g; Saturated Fat: 3g; Cholesterol: 138mg; Carbohydrates: 8g; Protein: 26g; Fiber: 2g; Sodium: 297mg

Chili-Lime Pork Loin

PREP TIME: 10 MINUTES, PLUS 1 HOUR TO MARINATE / **COOK TIME:** 30 MINUTES / **SERVES** 4 / 400°F

Marinating pork loin makes it extremely tender, and the combination of chili powder and lime in this one will give the meat a spicy, bold kick.

DAIRY-FREE

1 tablespoon lime juice
1 tablespoon olive oil, plus more for spraying
½ tablespoon soy sauce
½ tablespoon chili powder
¼ tablespoon minced garlic
1 pound boneless pork tenderloin

1. In a large zip-top plastic bag, mix together the lime juice, olive oil, soy sauce, chili powder, and garlic and mix well. Add the pork, seal, and refrigerate for at least 1 hour or overnight.

2. Spray a fryer basket lightly with olive oil.

3. Shake off any excess marinade from the pork and place it in the fryer basket.

4. Air fry for 15 minutes. Flip the tenderloin over and cook until the pork reaches an internal temperature of at least 145°F an additional 5 minutes. If necessary, continue to cook in 2- to 3-minute intervals until it reaches the proper temperature.

5. Let the tenderloin rest for 10 minutes before cutting into slices and serving.

Make it Gluten-Free: Soy sauce is normally made with wheat, but gluten-free soy sauce is readily available at grocery stores. Read labels carefully to be sure they are gluten-free.

Serve It With: Crispy Breaded Bell Pepper Strips are the ideal side dish to complete a satisfying, Southwestern-inspired meal.

Per Serving

Calories: 155; Total Fat: 6g; Saturated Fat: 2g; Cholesterol: 45mg; Carbohydrates: 1g; Protein: 23g; Fiber: <1g; Sodium: 182mg

Sweet and Spicy Pork Chops

PREP TIME: 10 MINUTES / **COOK TIME:** 15 MINUTES / **SERVES** 4 / 370°F

Pork is the most commonly consumed red meat in the world, but it is important to choose the right cut if you want to decrease the fat content. Pick lean pork loin chops and trim off any visible fat to keep this protein as heart healthy as possible.

DAIRY-FREE

GLUTEN-FREE

1 tablespoon olive oil, plus more for spraying
3 tablespoons brown sugar
½ teaspoon cayenne pepper
½ teaspoon garlic powder
½ teaspoon salt
¼ teaspoon freshly ground black pepper
4 thin boneless pork chops, trimmed of excess fat

1. Spray a fryer basket lightly with olive oil.

2. In a small bowl, mix together the brown sugar, 1 tablespoon of olive oil, cayenne pepper, garlic powder, salt, and black pepper.

3. Coat each pork chop with the marinade, shaking them to remove any excess, and place in the fryer basket in a single layer. You may need to cook them in batches.

4. Air fry for 7 minutes. Flip the pork chops over and brush with more marinade. Cook until the chops reach an internal temperature of 145°F, an additional 5 to 8 minutes.

Pair It With: Serve with Green Beans and New Potatoes for a balanced, hearty meal.

Per Serving

Calories: 188; Total Fat: 8g; Saturated Fat: 2g; Cholesterol: 55mg; Carbohydrates: 10g; Protein: 23g; Fiber: <1g; Sodium: 504mg

Breaded Italian Pork Chops

PREP TIME: 10 MINUTES / **COOK TIME:** 15 MINUTES / **SERVES** 4 / 370°F

The ingredients in Italian dry dressing mix usually include herbs like oregano, rosemary, thyme, and basil that bring a wonderful aroma and flavor whenever it's used. Keeping packets of the mix on hand allows you to marinate or season foods in mere minutes.

DAIRY-FREE

Olive oil
2 eggs, beaten
¼ cup whole-wheat bread crumbs
1 envelope zesty Italian dressing mix
4 thin boneless pork chops, trimmed of excess fat
Salt
Freshly ground black pepper

1. Spray a fryer basket lightly with olive oil.

2. Place the eggs in a shallow bowl.

3. In a separate shallow bowl, mix together the bread crumbs and Italian dressing mix.

4. Season the pork chops with salt and pepper. Coat the pork chops in the egg, shaking off any excess. Dredge them in the bread crumb mixture.

5. Place the pork chops in the fryer basket in a single layer and spray lightly with olive oil. You may need to cook them in batches.

6. Air fry for 7 minutes. Flip the pork chops over, lightly spray with olive oil, and cook until they reach an internal temperature of at least 145°F, an additional 5 to 8 minutes.

Pair It With: Serve these chops with Parmesan Green Beans for a filling meal bursting with Italian flavors.

Per Serving

Calories: 194; Total Fat: 7g; Saturated Fat: 2g; Cholesterol: 148mg; Carbohydrates:

6g; Protein: 27g; Fiber: 1g; Sodium: 691mg

Pork and Ginger Meatball Bowl

PREP TIME: 15 MINUTES / **COOK TIME:** 15 MINUTES / **SERVES** 4 / 390°F

Meatballs make a wonderful appetizer or main dish, but they're hard to fit into your diet when made with fatty meats. Using lean ground pork means you can keep these meatballs in your regular rotation. Ground ginger adds a spicy bite, while the gingerol it provides has antioxidant and anti-inflammatory properties.

DAIRY-FREE

Olive oil
2 pounds lean ground pork
2 eggs, beaten
1 cup whole-wheat panko bread crumbs
1 green onion, thinly sliced
2 teaspoons soy sauce
2 teaspoons minced garlic
½ teaspoon ground ginger
2 cups cooked rice noodles (cooked according to package directions)
1 cup peeled and shredded carrots
1 cup peeled and thinly sliced cucumber
1 cup light Asian sesame dressing

1. Spray a fryer basket lightly with olive oil.

2. In a large bowl, mix together the pork, eggs, bread crumbs, green onion, soy sauce, garlic, and ginger.

3. Using a small cookie scoop, form 24 meatballs.

4. Place the meatballs in a single layer in the fryer basket. Lightly spray meatballs with olive oil. You may need to cook the meatballs in batches.

5. Air fry until the meatballs reach an internal temperature of at least 145°F, 10 to 15 minutes, shaking the basket every 5 minutes for even cooking.

6. To assemble the bowls, place ½ cup rice noodles, ¼ cup carrots, and ¼ cup cucumber in 4 bowls. Drizzle each bowl with ¼ cup sesame dressing and top with 6 meatballs.

Per Serving

Calories: 642; Total Fat: 21g; Saturated Fat: 5g; Cholesterol: 213mg; Carbohydrates: 59g; Protein: 56g; Fiber: 5g; Sodium: 1,304mg

Hawaiian Pork Sliders

PREP TIME: 15 MINUTES / **COOK TIME:** 15 MINUTES / **SERVES** 4 / 370°F

The combination of pineapple and pork is beloved in Hawaiian culture. The flavors blend and balance out perfectly, and the sweetness of the pineapple means you don't need to add any additional sugary sauces. When you use an air fryer, they are cooked consistently every time.

DAIRY-FREE

Olive oil
½ cup crushed pineapple, drained
1 pound lean ground pork
1 teaspoon Worcestershire sauce
½ teaspoon garlic powder
½ teaspoon salt
½ teaspoon freshly ground black pepper
Pinch of cayenne pepper
8 whole-wheat slider buns

1. Spray a fryer basket lightly with olive oil.

2. In a large bowl, mix together the pineapple, pork, Worcestershire sauce, garlic powder, salt, and pepper.

3. Form the mixture into 8 patties.

4. Place the patties in the fryer basket in a single layer and spray lightly with olive oil. You may need to cook them in batches.

5. Air fry for 7 minutes. Flip the patties over, lightly spray with olive oil, and cook until the patties reach an internal temperature of at least 145°F, an additional 5 to 8 minutes.

6. Place the cooked patties on the slider buns and serve.

Make It Lower Calorie: One easy way to save calories is to eat your slider patty in a lettuce wrap instead of on a bun.

Pair It With: For an entirely hand-held meal, serve the sliders with Spicy Corn on the Cob.

Per Serving

Calories: 361; Total Fat: 8g; Saturated Fat: 2g; Cholesterol: 60mg; Carbohydrates: 42g; Protein: 32g; Fiber: 6g; Sodium: 786mg

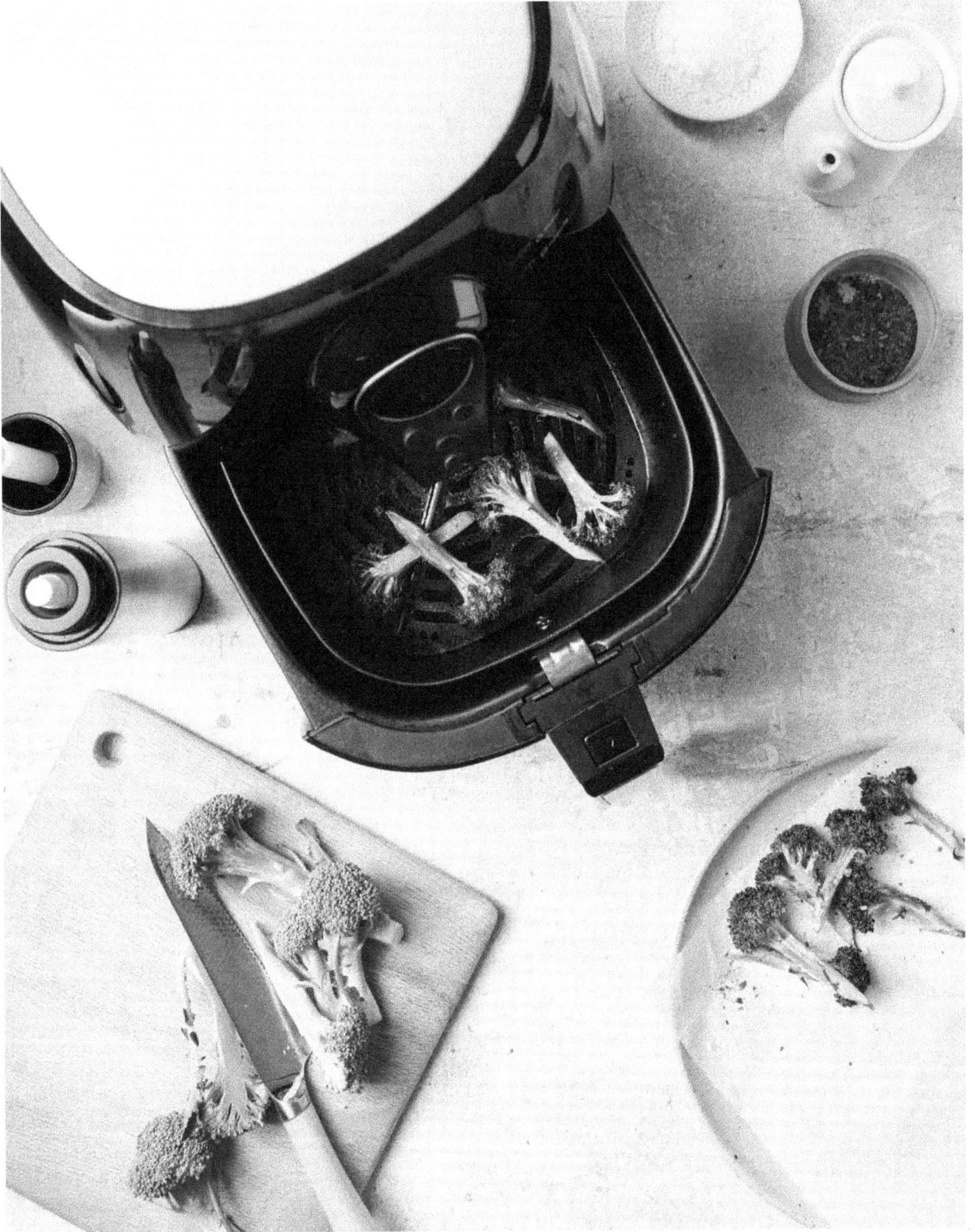

Measurement Conversions

	US Standard	US Standard (ounces)	Metric (approximate)
Volume Equivalents (Liquid)	2 tablespoons	1 fl. oz.	30 mL
	¼ cup	2 fl. oz.	60 mL
	½ cup	4 fl. oz.	120 mL
	1 cup	8 fl. oz.	240 mL
	1½ cups	12 fl. oz.	355 mL
	2 cups or 1 pint	16 fl. oz.	475 mL
	4 cups or 1 quart	32 fl. oz.	1 L
	1 gallon	128 fl. oz.	4 L
Volume Equivalents (Dry)	⅛ teaspoon		0.5 mL
	¼ teaspoon		1 mL
	½ teaspoon		2 mL
	¾ teaspoon		4 mL
	1 teaspoon		5 mL
	1 tablespoon		15 mL
	¼ cup		59 mL
	⅓ cup		79 mL
	½ cup		118 mL
	⅔ cup		156 mL
	¾ cup		177 mL
	1 cup		235 mL
	2 cups or 1 pint		475 mL
	3 cups		700 mL
	4 cups or 1 quart		1 L
	½ gallon		2 L
	1 gallon		4 L
Weight Equivalents	½ ounce		15 g
	1 ounce		30 g
	2 ounces		60 g
	4 ounces		115 g
	8 ounces		225 g

12 ounces		340 g
16 ounces or 1 pound		455 g

	Fahrenheit (F)	Celsius (C) (Approximate)
	250°F	120°C
	300°F	150°C
	325°F	180°C
Oven Temperatures	375°F	190°C
	400°F	200°C
	425°F	220°C
	450°F	230°C

www.ingramcontent.com/pod-product-compliance
Lightning Source LLC
Chambersburg PA
CBHW080621030426
42336CB00018B/3037